WILLIAM J. RYAN, Ph. D.
Speech Pathologist

THE ARTIFICIAL LARYNX HANDBOOK

THE ARTIFICIAL LARYNX HANDBOOK

Editors

Shirley J. Salmon, Ph.D.
Speech Pathologist
Veterans Administration Hospital
Kansas City, Missouri

Lewis P. Goldstein, Ph.D.
Speech Pathologist
Veterans Administration Hospital
Gainesville, Florida

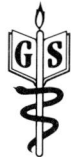

Grune & Stratton
A Subsidiary of Harcourt Brace Jovanovich, Publishers
New York   San Francisco   London

© **1978 by Grune & Stratton, Inc.**
All rights reserved. No part of this publication
may be reproduced or transmitted in any form or
by any means, electronic or mechanical, including
photocopy, recording, or any information storage
and retrieval system, without permission in
writing from the publisher.

Grune & Stratton, Inc.
111 Fifth Avenue
New York, New York 10003

Distributed in the United Kingdom by
Academic Press, Inc. (London) Ltd.
24/28 Oval Road, London NW 1

Library of Congress Catalog Number 78-13805
International Standard Book Number 0-8089-1111-2

Printed in the United States of America

Contents

Foreword	vii
Preface	ix
Contributors	xi
Section I Philosophy	**1**
1. Why Not Both? Marshall J. Duguay, Ph.D.	3
2. The Artificial Larynx: Pro and Con Lewis P. Goldstein, Ph.D.	11
3. Indications for the Use of Artificial Larynx Devices William R. Berry, Ph.D.	17
Section II Attitudes	**25**
4. Listener Judgments of Artificial Larynx Speech Lewis P. Goldstein, Ph.D.	27

5. Attitudes of Speech Pathologists and Otolaryngologists
    About Artificial Larynges
        William R. Berry, Ph.D.
	35

6. Patients Talk Back Shirley J. Salmon, Ph.D.	43

	Section III **Artificial Larynx Devices**	**55**
7.	**The Artificial Larynx: Past and Present** Eric D. Blom, Ph.D.	57
8.	**Analyzing Artificial Electronic Larynx Speech** Howard B. Rothman, Ph.D.	87
	Section IV **Treatment and Conclusions**	**113**
9.	**Approaches to Treatment**	115
	Part A William R. Berry	115
	Part B Eric D. Blom	118
	Part C Marshall J. Duguay	122
	Part D Lewis P. Goldstein	127
	Part E Howard B. Rothman	130
	Part F Shirley J. Salmon	137
10.	**Looking Ahead** Shirley J. Salmon	145
	Audio-Cassette Tape Outline	149
	Index	151

Foreword

The contributors to this volume provide information which has been sorely lacking in the rehabilitation literature of the laryngectomee. I first started my training in speech pathology in the early 1950s under Professor Warren Gardner, founder of the International Association of Laryngectomees (IAL). At that time the pendulum of rehabilitation for the laryngectomee was swinging away from predominant use of the artificial larynx, toward making both laryngectomized patients and the professionals aware that esophageal speech was possible for many. For the next 15 to 20 years, speech clinicians carried the torch for esophageal speech and neglected—in many cases, shunned—the artificial larynx. We saw the spawning of workshops that were sponsored by the Office of Vocational Rehabilitation (OVR) under the direction of Dr. Nathanial Levin, otolaryngologist. Then the American Cancer Society sponsored "voice institutes" under the leadership of the IAL and speech pathologists. Both the workshops and voice institutes were aimed primarily at training professionals to teach esophageal speech.

This book is important, not in directing the pendulum back to the artificial larynx, but in highlighting the total communication needs of the laryngectomized patient. The philosophy that is expressed here makes clear that the artificial larynx should not be considered when esophageal speech has failed, but should be introduced at the very beginning stages of the laryngectomee's communication training. The need to simultaneously teach both esophageal speech and the use of instruments is stressed. Furthermore, as the patient develops skill in utilizing both methods of speech in all types of demanding communication environments, he or she will be able to choose effectively and in an informed manner the best procedure for the particular situation. All members of the rehabilitation team (medical, nursing, social work, psychology, speech pathology, and family) need to be acquainted with the total range of communication possibilities for the laryngectomized patient. This comprehensive book on artificial larynges and their use fills a previously unmet need. It is for these reasons that *The Artificial Larynx Handbook* makes a valuable contribution.

William M. Diedrich, Ph.D.
Professor, Hearing and Speech Department
University of Kansas Medical Center
Kansas City, Kansas

Preface

Most of us are willing to acknowledge that much of what occurs in this world is neither totally right nor totally wrong. Yet in our everyday experiences we often function as if we believe otherwise. For example, a philosophical statement such as, "Given adequate knowledge, the larynegectomized person has the right to choose his method or methods of alaryngeal communication," implies that more than one way of communication can be right. Conversely, statements such as, "I'm really eager to help you learn how to talk. If it doesn't work out, you can always use the artificial larynx," implies there is only one right way to speak. The last quoted statement is representative of how speech-language pathologists and other professionals in the field have been talking for many years about artificial larynx speech. American Cancer Society literature, textbooks, and articles written by speech pathologists and otolaryngologists—or simply talking with a group of laryngectomees from almost anywhere in the country—verifys that this is the case.

Pendulums do swing, however, and a few people throughout the country are beginning to think and talk about artificial larynx speech in more accepting ways. A new philosophy toward use of artificial larynx devices is developing, and along with it the recognition that counseling and treatment procedures need to be altered accordingly.

The idea of a book about artificial larynx speech was first conceived in February 1977, following a workshop on artificial larynx devices which was sponsored by the Veterans Administration Regional Medical Education Center and held in Birmingham, Alabama. The need for this workshop was no doubt justified on the basis of statistics taken from several sources published and distributed by the American Cancer Society. In the June 1977 *IAL*

Newsletter it was reported that between 30,000 and 40,000 laryngectomees are now living in the United States. In the *1977 Cancer Facts and Figures*, it was estimated that cancer of the larynx is diagnosed in 9,200 new cases each year, and that it causes 3,350 deaths annually. When we consider these facts in conjunction with the knowledge that many laryngectomees do not develop serviceable esophageal speech, the reasons for having a workshop about artificial larynges become obvious.

Staff speakers at the workshop were selected because of their daily contact with laryngectomees and their original research relating to artificial larynx devices. They began by presenting information in a cautious and sometimes defensive manner. Participants, representing only a handful of speech pathologists who could have attended, at first seemed skeptical and occasionally even hostile. However, during the intervening hours of the workshop, many soul-searching discussions were held among staff and participants. Biases about artificial larynges gradually seemed to dissolve and newer, more positive thoughts about artificial larynx speech began to emerge. It was after reflecting upon the outcome of the workshop that the need for a book about artificial larynges became apparent.

The Artificial Larynx Handbook and accompanying audio-cassette tape presents a composite of information concerning artificial larynges and artificial larynx speech. Some of the information was provided at the workshop in Birmingham and elsewhere; some of it has not been presented before; and all of it is appearing for the first time here in published form.

The information will be of interest to anyone concerned with the rehabilitation of laryngectomees. More specifically, we believe it will be helpful to individuals directly involved with teaching alaryngeal communication. Our enthusiasm for presenting information about these topics, and our convictions that have stemmed from such information, may cause us to seem over-zealous. This is not our intent; rather, we hope that the content will be enlightening and cause introspection and reconsideration of previously established attitudes. The book was not written to promote the idea that one type of alaryngeal communication is right and another type is wrong. It was written to encourage professionals to reexamine their attitudes concerning artificial larynx devices and to seriously consider that much of what occurs in the world is neither totally right nor totally wrong.

In the accompanying tape cassette, there are examples of good speech from each commercially available artificial larynx. Also demonstrated are treatment procedures for achieving range of proficiency, speech projection, on–off tuning, use of paired words, coordination of speech and sound, attenuation of sound, placement, and pitch changes.

Shirley J. Salmon
Lewis P. Goldstein

CONTRIBUTORS

William R. Berry, Ph.D.
    Chief, Audiology & Speech Pathology Service
    V. A. Hospital
    Memphis, Tennessee

    Adjunct Associate Professor Speech Pathology
    Memphis State University
    Memphis, Tennessee

    Adjunct Assistant Professor of Neurology
    University of Tennessee Center for Health Sciences
    Memphis, Tennessee

Eric D. Blom, Ph.D.
    Chief, Audiology & Speech Pathology Service
    V. A. Hospital
    Indianapolis, Indiana

    Adjunct Associate Professor
    Department of Audiology & Speech Science
    Purdue University
    West Lafayette, Indiana

    Adjunct Associate Professor
    Department of Audiology & Speech Science
    Ball State University
    Muncie, Indiana

Marshall J. Duguay, Ph.D.
  Professor, Communication Disorders
  State University of New York
  College at Buffalo
  Buffalo, New York

Lewis P. Goldstein, Ph.D.
  Speech Pathologist
  V. A. Hospital
  Gainesville, Florida

  Adjunct Assistant Professor
  Institute for Advanced Study of the Communication Processes, and
    Department of Speech
  University of Florida
  Gainesville, Florida

Howard B. Rothman, Ph.D.
  Associate Professor
  Institute for Advanced Study of the Communication Processes, and
    Department of Speech
  University of Florida
  Gainesville, Florida

Shirley J. Salmon, Ph.D.
  Speech Pathologist
  V. A. Hospital
  Kansas City, Missouri

  Associate Professor
  Hearing and Speech Department
  University of Kansas Medical Center
  Kansas City, Kansas

THE ARTIFICIAL LARYNX HANDBOOK

Section I

PHILOSOPHY

For many years the use of the artificial larynx has been recommended only when all other speech rehabilitation measures failed. Fortunately such an attitude is changing. This section presents the philosophy that esophageal speech and artificial larynx speech should be learned and used simultaneously. Both the advantages and disadvantages of artificial larynges are discussed, as well as practical approaches for their use.

Marshall J. Duguay, Ph.D

1.
Why Not Both?

When I began working with laryngectomy patients back in the late 1950s, I little dreamed that I would ever write a chapter dealing with the artificial larynx. Like so many beginning professional workers in many different fields, I had a well-developed philosophy regarding just about everything. Nearly twenty years later I readily admit that most of those well-developed philosophies are still being developed. Usually this continuing development has resulted in better clinical service for the communicatively impaired. I realize I have made many mistakes, but I would like to believe that although I may have fallen, at least I fell forward.

I began working with laryngectomees in one of the world's most renowned cancer research centers, Roswell Park Memorial Institute. In those early days I knew what was best for my laryngectomy cases—and that excluded the use of the artificial larynx. Fortunately, my laryngectomy cases taught me differently. Unfortunately, my change was gradual. If the reader holds to the philosophy of not using artificial larynx devices, one of the primary reasons for writing this chapter is to change that point of view quickly. We may have performed a disservice in the past to some laryngectomees who looked to us for help in restoring their communication skills. It is within our power to deal more realistically and effectively with alaryngeal communication in the present and in the future. However, doing so may mean revising or changing some of our current beliefs.

COMMUNICATION

Fisher[1] writes, "The one form of communication which people use most effectively in interpersonal relationships is speech. With it, they give form to their innermost thoughts—their dreams, ambitions, sorrows and joys; without it, they are reduced to animal noises and unintelligible gestures. In a real sense, speech is the key to human existence." This is a powerful statement, and one not to be taken lightly. Its full impact probably is realized by the newly laryngectomized patient as he tries to write on his "magic slate" or convey a message to an attending nurse, doctor, or family member as they stand by with blank faces and try to feign comprehension. He has been *cut off* literally as well as figuratively from those around him.

The importance of the basic human need for communication must be appreciated by the speech pathologist, surgeon, physician, nurse, family member, friend, and other laryngectomees. There is a potential for harm when someone imposes his standard for verbal communication upon a new laryngectomee. We must not lose sight of the fact that it is communication that is important and not necessarily the manner of speaking. We do not fail as speech pathologists, nor do we fail as surgeons, nurses, or spouses if the laryngectomee does not use esophageal speech. Esophageal speech, in and of itself, is not necessarily the best or even the most desirable method of speaking after laryngectomy for some individuals. Those of us who come in contact with large numbers of laryngectomees can attest to the high prevalence of esophageal speakers who have failed to develop acceptable esophageal speech. Many are barely intelligible, have poor quality, and exhibit reduced intensity. They may employ extraneous and distracting body movements, facial grimaces, tracheal stoma blasts, or have audible "klunks" when taking air into the esophagus. They are—in spite of the presence of esophageal sound—extremely poor communicators. And poor postlaryngectomy speech communication is almost always an unnecessary and unfortunate condition to impose on a laryngectomized individual. It is also a condition which we can directly influence and control, beginning with our attitude and our philosophy toward alaryngeal speech.

THE PATIENT'S SATISFACTION

An important factor that must be considered is the satisfaction of the laryngectomee himself. A person talks primarily to meet needs and to control the environment. If communication needs can be met by using esophageal speech, a pneumatic artificial larynx, an electronic artificial larynx, surgically restored speech, or any combination of these methods, then and only then is *communication rehabilitation* complete. An excellent esophageal voice or excellent artificial larynx speech is of limited value if the person using it is dissatisfied. The way in which a given individual reacts determines whether or not a problem exists. Adjustment, for the most part, is achieved from within and not from without. This means that the laryngectomee must be satisfied with the way he speaks. Therefore he has a right to be involved in determining what method of speech is most satisfactory for him.

An important role of the professional should be to involve the patient actively in making realistic decisions about his method of communication. It should be remembered that our comments and our reactions as the speech pathologist, surgeon, or nurse have a profound influence on the patient. When you tell a laryngectomee to "Throw away that damn speaker and use an esophageal voice," or when you say "Well, if you can't learn to talk with an esophageal voice, you can always resort to an artificial larynx device," you are imposing your values, your biases, and your prejudices on him. Is that what is really intended? Or do you want the individual to accept his new way of communicating? Are you honestly trying to meet his communication needs or are you trying to meet yours?

If you cast the use of an artificial larynx into a negative light, such as sounding like a robot, a last resort, or something available for failures, you perform a real disservice to the patient. It is almost impossible to get a laryngectomee to accept an artificial larynx device and sometimes even to try one if he has been programmed against it. And for the most part, you are the one responsible for that programming.

FAILURE TO DEVELOP ESOPHAGEAL SPEECH

We know from the literature that large numbers of laryngectomees do not develop an acceptable esophageal voice. For example, Putney[2] reported that 38 percent of 440 patients failed to develop an esophageal voice. Gardner and Harris[3] suggested that 40 percent of laryngectomees do not acquire intelligible esophageal speech. Horn[4] found in his survey of 3,366 laryngectomees that about 36 percent did not develop serviceable esophageal speech. Martin[5] estimated that less than 50 percent of the laryngectomized population acquire adequate or socially acceptable esophageal speech. King, Fowlks, and Pierson,[6] reporting on 88 of their patients, said that 57.4 percent did not develop esophageal speech. If we add to these figures the laryngectomees who mistakenly believe that they have developed a good esophageal voice, the percentages become greater.

In our efforts to please esophageal speakers, or to avoid hurting their feelings, our silent approbation inadvertently reinforces some poor speakers into believing that they are good speakers. Surely, this is not our intent. Those who know large numbers of laryngectomees can easily name the few excellent speakers, for they are the exception and not the rule. In addition, much of the published research in the area of esophageal speech has been misleading and helped to distort our objectivity concerning esophageal speech; for the most part it was conducted by using the best esophageal speakers. Unfortunately, excellent esophageal speakers are a very small minority out of all esophageal speakers.

The implication of course is not that artificial larynx speech is superior to esophageal speech. In some cases esophageal speech is unquestionably superior, and in other cases artificial larynx speech is superior for the individual. If this truth is accepted, then it surely leads to the realization that there is a better way to approach alaryngeal voice therapy than simply in a single-track fashion.

A DUAL TRACK

Why, instead of either esophageal speech or an artificial larynx, can it not be both? Why can't a laryngectomee work on both esophageal speech and artificial larynx speech? Why can't he develop both methods of alaryngeal speech—each to their fullest extent? When we consider the number of hours devoted to esophageal voice training, how does the number of hours spent on artificial larynx speech compare? You likely have a subjective number of hours in mind, and the objective findings of Goldstein and Salmon reported in subsequent chapters will confirm the correctness or incorrectness of your "guesstimate." In most training situations the artificial larynx device is presented; a few brief instructions are given, mostly on how to turn it on and off and where to place it; and the client is sent away to attempt to communicate with it as best he can. He uses the device poorly because he was taught poorly, if at all. Listeners understandably react negatively because the result is poor speech. Then as the individual perceives their negative reactions, he reacts accordingly.

As professionals, we have contributed to this unfortunate and unnecessary situation. What we should be doing is teaching esophageal speech and artificial larynx speech simultaneously. The individual, a few days after surgery, can once again bridge the differences and distances that separate him from other human beings. In fact, several devices, with or without modifications, can be used almost immediately after surgery. One can readily appreciate this advantage for an illiterate laryngectomee. The use of such a device by an inpatient can certainly facilitate communication with the medical and nursing staff. A recent experience by a laryngectomee patient of mine illustrates this. He pushed the call button on his bedside stand to summon a nurse and she dutifully responded by asking "Can I help you?" However, she asked it from the nursing station over the intercom.

The laryngectomee can use an artificial larynx to talk with his children and family. He can tell his wife he loves her. When the telephone rings, he no longer has to tap once for yes and twice for no, but can actually talk to the party on the other end. Another important reason for using such a device is that it may enable a person to return to work, a status which realizes economic as well as emotional benefits. In short, the patient can once again feel like a needed and contributing human being. He does not have to use his "comic cartoon" magic slate to answer a question that was asked five sentences earlier in a one-sided conversation. How unfair it would be for us to deny him this dignity.

THE ARTIFICIAL LARYNX AS AN AID TO ESOPHAGEAL SPEECH ACQUISITION

As the patient learns to use the artificial larynx effectively, he can also commence working on esophageal speech. I have never heard of a case or seen a published report indicating that the use of an artificial larynx negated the acquisition of esophageal speech. As a matter of fact, the use of an artificial device concurrent with esophageal voice training may even facilitate the development of better esophageal speech.

It is obvious that people want to talk. Many laryngectomees want to talk so badly that they end up doing just that—talking badly. They begin using their limited esophageal speech for all speaking situations and, as a result of this practice, reinforce all of the negative aspects of their developing esophageal speech. It is generally easier to "just talk" than to concentrate and drill on the isolated tasks which contribute to speaking effectiveness. In a theoretical 16-hour "talk day," the bulk of speech behavior is directed toward communication and not to controlled practice. The result is a great deal of time devoted to using poor speech.

It seems reasonable to suggest that if one uses the device for communication and only practices "perfect" esophageal speech, the behavior reinforced will be a higher level of esophageal speech proficiency. I can attest to the effectiveness of the approach with laryngectomy patients who were air swallowers, rather than inhalers or injectors, and with pharyngeal speakers. Both types of problem case were switched to more appropriate methods of air intake for phonation. In order to facilitate the switch, they were instructed to use the device whenever they talked and to practice only the correct method of air intake for phonation. The use of a device was most effective in breaking the established faulty habits of swallowing and pharyngeal speech that formerly were present.

In addition, the use of a device reduces tension and anxiety which in turn can afford a better tonus in the region of the neo-glottis. We know that some anxiety can enhance learning but we also know that too much anxiety affects motor-skill learning. We have all seen the tension, effort, and struggle behavior exhibited by our anxious patients trying vainly to load air past a pharyngo-esophageal segment locked in tonic contraction. The harder they try, the more they fail, and a vicious cycle is established. If they used a device, they would no longer *have* to learn to talk and, as a result of this reduced anxiety, they might very well be able to learn esophageal phonation.

The use of a device during esophageal voice therapy sessions enables the patient to ask questions or request clarification from the clinician and thus to develop a better understanding of specific behavioral objectives. The importance of communication between teacher and pupil is basic to the learning process.

In addition to these important benefits, the use of a device greatly expands "communication time" per day and thus provides a greater opportunity to practice consonant articulation, the single most important factor affecting intelligibility. Articulation training which is provided to the artificial larynx user includes attention to generating sufficient intra-oral pressure for maximum consonant production, as well as attention to voicing and voiceless contrasts. These skills are important for the intelligibility of both artificial larynx and esophageal speech. The tendency of many laryngectomees who are learning only esophageal speech is to avoid speaking situations, or certainly to minimize them. They often avoid speaking because of the potential for failure and because no one tolerates repeated failures very well. Using a device contraindicates this avoidance, encourages communication experience, prevents social withdrawal, and provides more opportunities to use and improve articulation skills. Again, the importance of communication and the patient's emotional well-being is apparent.

OPTIONS

The laryngectomee can be taught to develop both methods of alaryngeal communication to their fullest extent. Then he has a number of options available to him. He does not have to settle for or accept any one method of speech since the two choices, esophageal speech and artificial larynx speech, began as equal and desirable alternatives. He can now choose to use either esophageal speech or artificial larynx speech. Preferably he will decide to use both. With both methods available, he can let the communication situation help determine which method to employ. He may, for example, elect to use his esophageal speech for general conversational activities and his artificial larynx speech to handle noisy environments such as a factory situation, riding in an automobile, or talking to a hard-of-hearing relative. Attempting to talk above competing background noise with esophageal speech is extremely demanding and intelligibility suffers. It is also much easier to use artificial larynx speech if a person is fatigued or ill.

An excellent esophageal speaker, who happens to be a physician and a director of the International Association of Laryngectomees,* relates an event that occurred in his speaking life. He received a telephone call in the early morning hours from a nurse in the emergency room at the hospital where he is affiliated. A patient of his had been brought in for emergency treatment and the nurse wanted to know how the case should be handled. Since he had just been aroused from a sound sleep and was dealing with a matter of grave importance, he found it very difficult to use his esophageal voice. (Many laryngectomees report that they need to "warm up" in the morning before they can depend on a good esophageal voice.) And he found that the harder he tried to talk (anxiety) the less success he experienced. He finally had to call his wife to the phone to talk for him. He reports vowing right then and there to go out and purchase an artificial larynx that same day, contrary to the wishes of his speech instructor. He did just that and expresses deep regret at not having had such a device from the beginning.

I can also remember an incident when a laryngectomee who could use only artificial larynx speech got up and went to work but left his "voice" home in a drawer. Neither of these incidents would have occurred if both methods were available to the laryngectomee. The person who wrote that silence is golden obviously knew nothing about laryngectomees.

It should be stressed that simultaneously working on both methods as the desirable goal prevents any stigma or negative feelings from becoming attached to one particular method. The person to benefit most from this approach is the person of greatest importance, the new laryngectomee.

One of the member clubs of the International Association of Laryngectomees, the Lost Chord Club of Cleveland, has for its motto, "Thank God for two voices in one lifetime." Perhaps it is time to change that motto to read, "Thank God for three voices in one lifetime." It does not have to be either/or; it can be both.

---

* JR Hall, M.D. 1977: personal communication.

REFERENCES

1. Fisher HB: Improving Voice and Articulation (ed 2). Boston, Houghton Mifflin, 1975, p 3
2. Putney EJ: Rehabilitation of the post-laryngectomized patient. Ann Otol Rhinol Laryngol 67:544–549, 1958
3. Gardner WN, Harris HE: Aids and devices for laryngectomees. Arch Otholaryngol 73:145–152, 1961
4. Horn D: Laryngectomee survey report. Eleventh Annual Meeting, International Association of Laryngectomees, Memphis, Tennessee, 1962
5. Martin H: Rehabilitation of the laryngectomee. Cancer 16:823–841, 1963
6. King PS, Fowlks EW, Pierson GA: Rehabilitation and adaptation of laryngectomy patients. Am J Phys Med 47:192–203, 1968

Lewis P. Goldstein, Ph.D.

2.
The Artificial Larynx: Pro and Con

The literature dealing with the speech of the laryngectomee is heavily biased toward esophageal speech training, ignoring the fact that at least one-third of the laryngectomized population cannot or does not use it. Early articles that discussed the availability of artificial larynges were also quick to include reasons why they should not be used. Even today many speech pathologists, otolaryngologists, and esophageal-speaking laryngectomees are only willing to discuss the disadvantages of the artificial larynx. Using the adage that nothing is all bad, both the advantages and disadvantages of the artificial larynx will be discussed in this chapter.

I have compiled, in separate lists, the twelve most frequent reasons which have appeared in the literature *for* and *against* the use of an artificial larynx. These lists are comprehensive though not complete, as they include only items that have been mentioned in the literature at least twice.

DISADVANTAGES OF THE ARTIFICIAL LARYNX

1. Produces an unacceptable sound.
2. Early use interferes with esophageal speech development.
3. Speech produced is unintelligible.
4. The instrument is a crutch.
5. Calls attention to the inability to speak normally.
6. Is a sign of defeat.
7. Requires the use of one hand.

8. Is bulky and awkward to handle.
9. Maintenance is expensive.
10. Mechanical breakdown makes the patient helpless.
11. Is awkward for casual remarks.
12. Patient does not think he is doing the talking.

Discussion of the Disadvantages

Some of these statements may or may not be valid. The following discussion of the twelve disadvantages analyzes the validity of each assertion.

1. The degree of unacceptability of the sound produced by an artificial larynx is related to the proficiency of the speaker. Listen to the range of proficiency on the accompanying cassette. With the poorer speakers, you will notice that you are more aware of the artificial sound than of what is being said. Conversely, with the better speakers you can attend to what they are saying and therefore you become aware of the artificial sound only to the extent that you know they are not using a laryngeal or esophageal voice.

2. The controversy as to whether or not the use of an artificial larynx interferes with esophageal speech development is still not resolved. Presently there is no data to substantiate either position. My own clinical experience, as well as that of some of my colleagues, has led me to conclude that immediate use of the artificial larynx does not interfere with learning esophageal speech. Diedrich and Youngstrom[1] state that "It is possible that the aid could speed up the learning of esophageal speech." Having some form of communication (other than writing and whispering) enables the new laryngectomee to relax and gain the necessary confidence to develop esophageal speech.

3. Speech produced with the artificial larynx is completely intelligible if the instrument is used correctly. As demonstrated on the cassette, an individual should be able to make himself easily understood. Proper usage of an artificial larynx can be taught and learned rather easily. However, individuals do need proper instruction, feedback, and considerable practice before they achieve effective intelligibility.

4 and **6.** Whether the artificial larynx is considered to be a crutch or a sign of defeat is related to how it is initially presented. If a laryngectomee is told that it is not the preferred method of talking, or that he can only use it for a specific period of time, his attitude toward the instrument will be negative.

5. The use of an artificial larynx does call attention to the inability to speak normally. But this is also true of an individual who whispers, uses sign language, or communicates through writing. To some degree this statement is also true for esophageal speakers, since all methods of alaryngeal speech sound different from speech produced with a normally functioning larynx.

7 through 10. One must fully agree with items 7 through 10 against the use of the artificial larynx. However, recent advances in technology, primarily due to the space age and its attendant need for miniaturization, have provided the means and technical knowledge to improve existing artificial larynges. However, given the dictates of economic pressures, improvements will be undertaken only with increased usage and acceptance of these devices by laryngectomees and their circle of listeners.

11 and **12.** Many laryngectomees have expressed dissatisfaction at having to reach for, place, and activate an artificial larynx for casual or one-word expressive remarks. Further, it has often been heard from laryngectomees that they do not feel as if they are actually speaking. These feelings or beliefs must be given serious consideration because they are generated by individuals with a real problem. However, I believe that the attitudes responsible for these negative expressions can be mitigated during the early stages of each laryngectomee's rehabilitation.

SUMMARY

It is obvious from the previous discussion that I have attempted to minimize the disadvantages of the artificial larynx. However, it is also evident that for many years these ideas have been put forth with little or no attempt to quantify or objectively analyze their validity. More recently the literature has reflected a change in attitude which has led to the appearance of reasons promoting the use of the artificial larynx.

ADVANTAGES OF THE ARTIFICIAL LARYNX

1. Useful in advanced age.
2. Useful in poor physical or mental health.
3. Useful when one fails to learn esophageal speech.
4. Permits prompt and immediate speech.
5. Better than living in silence and seclusion.
6. Easily learned.
7. Better than writing.
8. Early return to work is possible.
9. Voice is more uniform than esophageal speech.
10. Volume is better than esophageal speech.
11. Easily understood over the telephone.
12. Is free from grimaces and stoma noise.

Discussion of the Advantages

Again, some of these statements may or may not be valid. The twelve advantages also are discussed here in their proper perspective.

1 through 3. Limiting the usefulness of the artificial larynx to individuals of certain ages or conditions of health is extremely shortsighted. All laryngectomized individuals should receive equal benefits. Each patient should be given an artificial larynx with proper instructions for its use, as well as the opportunity to learn esophageal speech. Making decisions solely on the basis of an individual's age or condition of health can lead to clinical error. Recently an 83-year-old laryngectomee was referred to a clinic for an artificial larynx. Because of his advanced age and poor health, his physician surmised that he couldn't learn esophageal speech. This individual learned to use an artificial larynx and then inquired about esophageal speech when he heard about it from associating with other laryngectomees. Within a three-week period this 83-year-old laryngectomee was using both esophageal and artificial larynx speech effectively. As stated previously, both methods should be introduced early to insure that some form of communication will be established.

4 through 7. A few individuals can learn to use the artificial larynx quite easily, thereby permitting prompt and immediate speech. However, the naive and irresponsible idea prevails among some clinicians that all they must do to teach artificial larynx speech is to give the laryngectomee the artificial larynx, instruct him in the proper placement of the instrument, and explain how to turn it on and off. Some people do learn artificial larynx speech easily, but most require time and proper instruction before they can learn to use it proficiently. Leaving an individual on his own to acquire the skills needed for the proper use of the artificial larynx leads to exaggeration of the mechanical aspects of artificial larynx speech, poor intelligibility, and considerable frustration on the part of both listener and speaker.

Everyone will probably agree that living in silence or having to communicate solely by writing is an unacceptable alternative. For this reason alone, each laryngectomee should be given an artificial larynx as soon after surgery as possible. For those clinicians who are not convinced, it is suggested that they try spending one or two days either in silence or in communicating only by writing.

8. Many laryngectomees must return to employment quickly for economic, social, and psychological reasons. Use of the artificial larynx provides them with a form of communication that is acceptable in most types of employment.

9 through 12. Advantages 9 through 12 are not guaranteed by virtue of using an artificial larynx. The advantageous features of using the artificial larynx—stability of sound, volume, intelligibility, and lack of grimacing and stoma noise—must be encouraged and sometimes taught to the laryngectomee.

CONCLUSION

Much of the reasoning responsible for generating the advantages and/or disadvantages of the artificial larynx is extremely subjective. Perhaps the most persuasive reason for making an artificial larynx available to all laryngectomized individuals, including those proficient in esophageal speech, has been provided by Lauder.[2] He describes three events involving laryngectomized patients in acute situations which precluded the use of esophageal speech. One person had an attack of pancreatitis and could not communicate with a physician by telephone; a second had a draining hypopharyngeal fistula which exuded copious secretions at each attempt to inject air for esophageal speech; and the third had not developed esophageal speech, and therefore could not communicate the fact that his wife was having a heart attack. These three cases admittedly are extreme, but they illustrate that when an available procedure is ignored, the effects can be significant.

Every laryngectomized individual should have an unbiased opportunity to judge the potential of using an artificial larynx as well as to judge other methods for developing adequate speech communication. The final decision should be based on the individual laryngectomee—his physical and mental state, and his circle of listeners.

REFERENCES

1. Diedrich WM, Youngstrom KA: Alaryngeal Speech. Springfield, Charles C Thomas, 1966, p 141
2. Lauder E: The laryngectomee and the artificial larynx—a second look. J Speech Hear Disord **35:**62–65, 1970

William R. Berry, Ph.D.

3.
Indications for the Use of Artificial Larynx Devices

In some respects there should be no need for this chapter. The need is real, unfortunately, because of ignorance and/or bias. Many clinicians, even experienced ones, are unsure about whether to issue artificial larynx devices. Some reasons for this are:

1. Students of speech pathology receive almost no training in artificial larynx devices.
2. Many speech pathologists have developed such a negative bias against the use of artificial larynges that to issue one is like admitting defeat.

We need to begin breaking down these barriers to proper clinical management of the laryngectomee.

TO USE OR NOT TO USE?

Whether or not to use an artificial larynx is A question, but not THE question, and certainly not the FIRST question. For some clinicians it is not even a question; they choose to ignore this avenue of treatment altogether.

"To use or not to use" implies that an a priori decision is made by someone. It should be that the someone is the patient, but many times this is unfortunately not the case. All too often the laryngectomee will begin therapy without knowing that he has some choices concerning his verbal communication. Therefore the laryngectomee is susceptible to the opinions of those to whom he has entrusted his future. It is vital that he be given every opportunity to control his destiny.

Information is the key. Either before or immediately after surgery, depending upon the opportunity for counseling, the speech pathologist should present the salient facts concerning the postoperative treatment. This should include all of the positive and negative aspects about both esophageal speech and artificial larynx speech. All of these factors should be considered in conjunction with the patient's physical and psychological status, education, and environment, as well as his personal, vocational, and social expectations. Only in this way will the patient be able to make an informed decision to use or not to use an artificial larynx.

A LOOK AT ALL THE ANGLES

What are some of the factors that should be presented to the patient so that he can adequately make his decision? First, the speech clinician should help to prevent the patient from being biased by other sources. The most well-intentioned clinician can be undermined by a surgeon, nurse, or other paraprofessional who cannot tolerate the sound of an artificial larynx. In-service education and close communication can build an understanding between rehabilitation team members (i.e., speech pathologist, surgeon, nurse, social worker, family) who must learn that candid negative comments will never serve the patient's well-being. Care also should be taken not to bias the prospective laryngectomee with a presurgical visit from a laryngectomee who may express opinions against the use of an artificial larynx. If the laryngectomee visitor exclusively uses esophageal speech, the patient indirectly can get the idea that this is the ultimate model. If possible, a visitor should be chosen who competently demonstrates the use of both esophageal speech and at least one type of artificial larynx speech.

At an appropriate time after surgery, the clinician should discuss with the patient the factors listed below. A discussion of these factors is appropriate for educating the patient and for helping him to objectify his ideas concerning esophageal speech and artificial larynx speech. Later decisions about when to use one method of communication or the other will be based on individual needs and limitations. An added benefit of using this list of factors for discussion purposes is that it can systematize the clinician's remarks and, in so doing, minimize the possibility of imposing bias into the counseling session.

1. Therapy time.
2. Neo-voice quality.
3. Use of hands.
4. Cost.

INDICATIONS FOR THE USE OF ARTIFICIAL LARYNX DEVICES

5. Overall loudness.
6. Power supply.
7. Production reliability.

During the discussion of these factors, the laryngectomized patient will learn that the development of a serviceable level of esophageal speech typically requires more time than the development of serviceable artificial larynx speech. It should be made clear to the patient that most artificial larynx devices sound more mechanical than esophageal speech. However, the quality of esophageal voice varies considerably among esophageal speakers. The patient will learn that with esophageal speech his hands can be totally free while speaking, whereas he will need to use at least one hand to operate an artificial larynx device. Another factor to be discussed is that speech with artificial larynx devices is generally louder than esophageal speech, and it is often better understood in noisy environments. For most laryngectomees the esophagus is more reliable as a power supply for speech than the mechanical aspects of an artificial larynx. Another factor to be discussed is cost. Learning to use an artificial larynx is generally less expensive than learning to use esophageal speech because the number of treatment sessions are fewer. However, on-going cost of battery replacement and maintenance repairs must be considered for artificial larynx speech. The patient should likewise be cautioned that there are times when esophageal speech is not reliable. Even good esophageal speakers may have difficulty speaking when they are fatigued or under stress.

All of these factors should be discussed in order to present a complete picture to the patient. With such a procedure the laryngectomee can participate in the decision-making process, which will probably result in a more personal commitment to treatment. Once the patient commits himself or makes a decision, the clinician should respect his choice and support it with professional fervor.

The laryngectomee's decision need not be made hastily. Actually it is important that, during the initial phase of treatment, the patient be given the opportunity to completely understand each factor. One way to accomplish this is to enter therapy with a "combined approach"; that is, letting the patient try to initiate esophageal sound as well as use a variety of artificial larynx devices. Early treatment should be low-key and any verbal success, no matter of what type, should be rewarded with much social praise.

Others have pointed out that early therapy need not be confined to exclusive use of either esophageal speech or artificial larynges, unless the patient has made such a decision after being presented with all the facts. Have you ever heard a statement like "Well, let's try to work on esophageal speech in the beginning of therapy, and if we seem to have trouble, we'll consider using an artificial larynx." I know that such statements are made because I used to make them, until I realized that a few patients who could not learn esophageal speech, for whatever reason, felt like failures when we "had to" rely on an artificial larynx device. Since I had refrained from an early introduction of artificial devices, it must have seemed to the laryngectomee like second-rate communication compared to esophageal speech.

The laryngectomee should never develop a feeling of inferiority from his clinician, certainly not if he has learned effective speech with an artificial larynx. Probably nothing in my career made me feel smaller than when one of my patients apologized to me for the quality of his speech after developing very proficient communication with an electronic larynx. He had tried to acquire esophageal sound for over three months as he communicated with a magic slate. At that point we decided to consider an artificial larynx. At the end of one week he was speaking fluently and intelligibly with an artificial larynx, but he despised the sound of his speech, which caused him to withdraw from communicative opportunities. I never was able to change his behavior. He continued to try to develop esophageal sound and finally achieved his goal. As soon as he could produce single syllables with esophageal speech, he returned his artificial larnyx to me. Almost 5½ years later, he speaks somewhat unintelligibly at the single-syllable level with esophageal speech and refuses to speak with a device. It was this patient who made me realize that my latent bias had caused his problems. Sharing my error perhaps will prevent others from making a similar error.

SPECIFIC INDICATIONS

I have emphasized that everything possible should be done to allow the patient to choose his own type of communication. I have also made no secret of my bias that the patient should try a number of different devices early in treatment to determine the best one for him. During this process, the clinician may be asked by the patient to offer a value judgment: for example, the patient may say, "Hey Doc, which one do you think I should use?"

Assuming that we clinicians are going to utilize a combined treatment approach (i.e., attempting to develop use of esophageal speech as well as use of an artificial larynx) we must offer guidance to assist the patient in his decision making. The ability to assist the patient implies adequate training and experience to make recommendations about the type of device that best fits the patient's communicative needs. Following are some factors to be considered when recommending one of the major types of devices.

Surgery

Some speech-language pathologists are demonstrating several different types of artificial larynges prior to surgery. The artificial larynx device that is selected by the patient preoperatively should be the one used postoperatively unless there are contraindications. A neck-type instrument or a pneumatic device is not indicated immediately following surgery whenever there is pain or tenderness in the neck or stoma regions. Consequently, an intra-oral electronic larynx should probably be the first aid recommended to the laryngectomee. An intra-oral electronic device should also be used if the patient develops a postoperative fistula; neck-type devices are contraindicated because the neck vibration may impede the closing of the fistula.

Hearing

Significant hearing impairment is a major obstacle for any laryngectomee, and it should affect his choice of device. Many patients report that some neck-type electronic larynges vibrate in a way that prevents adequate auditory monitoring of their self-generated speech signal. Utilization of a neck-type device on the cheek, occasionally used with some patients, also will be difficult because the sound is conducted directly via the bones into the cochlea, which significantly impedes auditory feedback. In each of these instances, several alternatives should be presented to the patient so that he can choose the one which permits the best self-monitoring.

Oral Habits and Abilities

Poor articulation habits or abilities are a negative factor in therapy no matter which device is selected. Some individuals find it difficult to articulate with an intra-oral tube. However, the tubes from the different devices vary in diameter. The tubes with thinner walls promote better intelligibility. Dentures, structural damage, dysarthria, or other factors impeding oral mobility also will have to be considered when choosing a proper aid. Oral hygiene, or lack thereof, is another factor to be considered since intra-oral tubing can become plugged or susceptible to bacterial growth.

Neck Tissue

A neck-type aid cannot be used if the neck tissue is a poor conductor of the vibratory signal. Obesity, tissue necrosis, scar tissue, pain, or combinations thereof may indicate the use of an intra-oral device. On occasion a laryngectomee may exhibit a dermal hypersensitivity reaction on the neck when using a neck-type aid and have to employ an intra-oral device, at least temporarily.

Stoma Phobia

There are laryngectomees who reject the use of pneumatic artificial larynx devices because they fear having the stoma covered. Even when they are counseled, their fears cannot be diminished. If this is the case, a neck-type or electronic intra-oral device should be offered as an alternative.

Dexterity

The ability to synchronize a number of movements with the hands is of course very important in the use of any type of artificial larynx device. If the laryngectomee has dexterity problems because of arthritis, motoric impairment, structural damage, and so on, patience is needed to determine the best artificial larynx device. If placement is difficult with a neck-type device, an intra-oral aid may be the solution. Manipulation of controls with some type of electronic larynx may be easier than with others. If manipulation of pitch control and the timing of signal initiation cannot be mastered, the pitch control mechanism can either be disconnected or ignored. Modifications can be made with some types of pneumatic aids so that only one hand is necessary or so that the stoma cup need not be lifted during speech. These modifications will lessen the dexterity requirements.

Environment

Immediate and long-range environmental needs may influence the patient's decision about which device to select. The laryngectomee should be informed of possible environmental problems. The attitude of family or friends also will have to be considered and the family should be counseled to support the choice of device. Mitigating factors, such as a family member's hearing loss, may indicate one type of aid for improved intelligibility even though it is not the patient's first choice. Other types of environmental factors include regular exposure to ambient noise, amount of telephone usage, and vocational constraints. Many times the patient and the clinician will have to try several types of artificial larynx devices to accommodate these various environmental factors.

Cost

The cost factor cannot be ignored since artificial larynx devices range from $25 to over $300. If third-party payment support is not available, then the price of the device may influence the choice.

Trial Aids

It is imperative that a stock of artificial larynx devices be available so that each patient can try different aids, weigh the factors mentioned, and make a practical and intelligent choice. If you do not have such a stock, get one! Perhaps a local service organization can be persuaded to purchase the needed devices.

SUMMARY

This information has been presented to help the clinician discuss artificial larynx devices intelligently when interacting with laryngectomee patients. It may cause some experienced individuals to reconsider their methods. Selection of the appropriate artificial larynx device is a challenge both to the patient and the clinician, who should work together as a team. The challenge can produce very positive communication rewards, and that's the name of the game.

Section II

ATTITUDES

The attitudes of several clinicians are presented to explore current practices concerning early usage of the artificial larynx in alaryngeal rehabilitation. Included in this section are studies concerning listeners' judgments of alaryngeal speech, and the opinions of speech pathologists and otolaryngologists about the use of artificial larynx devices. In conclusion, and of utmost importance, the experiences of artificial larynx speakers themselves are discussed.

Lewis P. Goldstein, Ph.D.

4.
Listener Judgments of Artificial Larynx Speech

How good is the artificial larynx for communication? How does it compare to esophageal speech? What do others think of speech produced with an artificial larynx? These and similar questions have been asked by many people in the field of speech pathology. The following studies have added to our knowledge of listener judgments of artificial larynx speech.

REVIEW OF THE RESEARCH

Hyman[1] compared listener preference, intelligibility, and physical measurements of esophageal speech, artificial larynx speech, and normal speech. Selection criteria for the alaryngeal subjects included at least six months usage of one method of speech and a level of effective speech as judged by the investigator and two assistants. All the artificial larynx speakers used a pneumatic type of appliance. Using college students to judge audio tape recordings of eight normal, eight esophageal, and eight artificial larynx speakers reading a word list and standard passage, these results were determined:

1. Artificial larynx speakers were always preferred in comparison to esophageal speakers.
2. Artificial larynx speakers were significantly louder than normal or esophageal speakers.
3. Artificial larynx speakers took less time than esophageal speakers but more time than normal speakers to read a standard passage.

4. Intelligibility of speech produced with the artificial larynx and with the esophageal method were not significantly different.

Similarly Crouse[2] compared listener preferences between esophageal speech and artificial larynx speech. However, she not only used an audio (tape recording) presentation, but also incorporated an audio-visual (sound-motion picture) presentation. Subject selection was based on the fact that each individual had used his method of postlaryngectomy speech for at least one year and was considered to be a good speaker as judged by the investigator. The artificial larynx speakers used pneumatic and electronic devices. Listeners consisted of an equal number of trained speech pathologists and nonprofessional people. Their task was to state a preference between five esophageal speakers and five artificial larynx speakers reading a standard passage. The stimuli were presented by both tape recordings and sound-motion pictures. The results indicated that esophageal speech was preferred over artificial larynx speech by both groups of judges under both types of stimulus conditions.

In an effort to determine differences in listeners, McCroskey and Mulligan[3] compared the intelligibility of esophageal and artificial larynx speech, as judged by three different groups of listeners. All subjects had used their method of speech for more than one year. Of the artificial larynx subjects, three used an electronic artificial larynx and two used a device involving the insertion of a tube in the mouth. A multiple-choice intelligibility word list was tape-recorded and played back to three groups of listeners: experienced speech pathologists, graduate speech students, and a group of naive listeners. Analysis of the data indicated that esophageal speech was more intelligible than artificial larynx speech to professional and student listeners. Conversely, naive listeners indicated higher intelligibility among artificial larynx speakers than among esophageal speakers.

Shames, Font, and Matthews[4] studied several variables that might be related to the learning of esophageal speech by alaryngeal patients. Of the 153 laryngectomized subjects, 118 were esophageal speakers and 35 were artificial larynx speakers. Most of the artificial larynx speakers used an electronic device. The only selection criteria was that the laryngectomee's speech training had been completed. Undergraduate students judged tape recordings of both a standard passage and isolated words. They determined word intelligibility, total time used in speaking, articulation accuracy, and surd-sonant errors of each speaker. Analysis of the data revealed that artificial larynx speakers read significantly faster than esophageal speakers. However, esophageal speakers were superior to artificial larynx speakers on word intelligibility. There were no significant differences between the two types of speakers in their sentence intelligibility.

Bennett and Weinberg[5] compared acceptability ratings of esophageal, artificial larynx, and normal speech. Since they were interested in determining acceptability of alaryngeal speech, they studied only proficient laryngectomized speakers and employed naive listeners. The artificial larynx subjects used different devices: one Western Electric 5A, two Western Electric 2A reed devices, and one Tokyo artificial larynx. Ratings of audio-tape samples of a standard passage revealed the following results.

1. Speech with the Tokyo artificial larynx was rated as more acceptable than speech with all other types of artificial larynges.
2. Esophageal speech was preferred over artificial larynx speech.
3. Alaryngeal speech was always judged as not normal.

Goldstein,[6] in the process of comparing psychological and nonpsychological variables between a group of esophageal and artificial larynx speakers, also compared their verbal communication proficiency. Selection criteria for the alaryngeal speakers were that they had completed treatment and used only one method of speaking. All the artificial larynx speakers used an electronic device. Ratings from speech pathologists were used to determine general verbal communication proficiency. All judgments were based on the speech pathologists' past experiences and were made from tape-recorded samples of everyday sentences. Statistical comparison indicated no significant difference between verbal communication proficiency of the two groups.

Kalb[7] compared the intelligibility of esophageal speech and artificial larynx speech produced by different speakers as well as by the same speaker. Five esophageal speakers, five artificial larynx speakers using electronic devices, and five laryngectomees using both methods of speech were selected and matched for proficiency. Kalb used 30 naive listeners to determine word intelligibility from audio-tape samples. Analysis of the data determined that there was no difference in intelligibility between esophageal and artificial larynx speech when each method was produced by the same speaker. However, esophageal speakers were more intelligible than artificial larynx speakers when the two groups of different speakers were compared.

Discussion

Table 4-1 summarizes the studies concerning listener judgments of artificial larynx speech compared to esophageal speech. Comparison of the results can become confusing and contradictory. One quickly becomes aware that our knowledge of listener judgment is far from complete. But why such conflicting results? Two possible explanations may be found through a discussion of the subjects and listeners used in the studies.

Bennett and Weinberg[5] suggested that the difference among the various

Table 4-1.
Summary of the Literature Pertaining to Listener Judgments of Artificial Larynx Speech as Compared to Esophageal Speech.

Study	Subjects	Listeners	Stimuli	Method	Question	Results
Hyman 1955	8 norms 8 Eso. 8 AL All Pn.	120 students	Standard passage Words	Audio	Preference Intelligibility	AL preferred Equal Intelligibility
Crouse 1962	5 Eso. 5 AL 2 Pn. 3 El.	12 professional 12 naive	Standard passage	Audio-visual Audio	Preference	Eso. preferred in all conditions
McCroskey and Mulligan 1963	5 Eso. 5 AL 2 Pn. 3 El.	10 professional 10 students 10 naive	Words	Audio	Intelligibility	Eso. more intelligible by professional judges AL more intelligible by naive judges
Shames, Font, and Matthews 1963	118 Eso. 35 AL 2 Pn. 33 El.	5 students	Standard passage Words	Audio	Proficiency Intelligibility	AL read faster Eso. better word intelligibility Equal sentence intelligibility

Table 4-1 (continued).

Study	Subjects	Listeners	Stimuli	Method	Question	Results
Bennett and Weinberg 1973	9 norms 5 Eso. 4 AL 3 Pn. 1 El.	37 naive	Standard passage	Audio	Acceptability	AL with Tokyo most acceptable Eso. more acceptable than other AL devices
Goldstein 1975	15 Eso. 15 AL All El.	6 professional	Sentences	Audio	Proficiency	Equal proficiency
Kalb 1977	5 Eso. 5 AL All El. 5 Both	30 naive	Words	Audio	Intelligibility	Equal intelligibility with those using both methods Eso. more intelligible between groups

Eso. = esophageal   Pn. = pneumatic device
AL = artificial larynx   El. = electronic device

studies may be a result of subject selection. All of the studies compared speakers who were post-treatment. However, the time span since the termination of treatment varied. The amount and type of treatment also may have varied both within and between groups. Goldstein[6] found that the average time of treatment for esophageal speakers was 18.10 hours, whereas artificial larynx speakers averaged 2.23 hours of treatment. Treatment should affect the proficiency and intelligibility of the speaker. Therefore, comparisons between a trained group of speakers and a relatively untrained group of speakers are likely to yield questionable results.

Attention should also be called to the type of instrument used by each subject. Some of Crouse's[2] speakers used an electronic device and others used a pneumatic device. Does comparing a group of esophageal speakers with a group of speakers using different types of devices (which we tend to lump together as artificial larynx speakers) tend to skew or bias the results? Further, is each artificial larynx speaker using the device that is most proficient for him, or is he using a device chosen solely on availability, economic feasibility, or biased professional recommendation? Possibly, a group of trained artificial larynx speakers using instruments that have been carefully selected to match their individual needs would reflect different results when compared to esophageal speakers.

In most studies no consideration is given to why the artificial larynx speakers use a device rather than esophageal speech. Have they had extensive surgery or radiation, making them unable to produce esophageal speech? Do they have other medical or psychological barriers precluding esophageal speech development? Many of the reasons that interfere with acquiring esophageal speech will also interfere with effective artificial larynx speech. Although these individuals are usually able to produce intelligible speech with an artificial larynx, can they be considered comparable to esophageal speakers who may not have secondary problems affecting their speech? Possibly not. The results of Kalb's study[7] indicate than when utilizing the same speaker for esophageal and artificial larynx speech, equal intelligibility results; but when utilizing different speakers for esophageal and artificial larynx speech, the two methods are not equally intelligible.

Another major consideration is the selection of listeners. McCroskey and Mulligan[3] used both speech pathologists and naive listeners, but they obtained different results from each group. This fact led them to conclude that intelligibility scores may be influenced by professional training or professional bias. Obviously we need more information about the individuals who are making the comparison between esophageal and artificial larynx speech. In order to properly evaluate the results of the studies cited here, it is necessary to know the extent of experience that the speech pathologist listeners had with alaryngeal speakers. Another important factor is the amount of direct experience they had with artificial larynx speakers. This information would help eliminate listeners who might have a bias toward esophageal speech. It also would be of interest to know if the group of naive listeners had ever known a laryngectomee and, if so, the type of speech the laryngectomee used. By knowing more about our listeners we may be able to give a more definite answer concerning judgments of alaryngeal speech.

SUMMARY

We have reviewed seven studies that compared esophageal speakers and artificial larynx speakers. Although the results of these studies do not agree, there are indications that artificial larynx speech has merit. It is also apparent that more information in this area is needed.

REFERENCES

1. Hyman M: An experimental study of artificial larynx and esophageal speech. J Speech Hear Disord 20:291–299, 1955
2. Crouse GP: An Experimental Study of Esophageal and Artificial Larynx Speech, thesis. Emory University, Atlanta, 1962
3. McCroskey R, Mulligan M: The relative intelligibility of esophageal speech and artificial larynx speech. J Speech Hear Disord 28:37–41, 1963
4. Shames GH, Font J, Matthews J: Factors related to speech proficiency of the laryngectomized. J Speech Hear Disord 28:273–287, 1963
5. Bennett S, Weinberg B: Acceptability ratings of normal, esophageal, and artificial larynx speech. J Speech Hear Res 16:608–615, 1973
6. Goldstein LP: A Study of the Relationship Between Adience–Abience Scale Scores and Judgments of Verbal Communication Proficiency of a Group of Esophageal Speakers and a Group of Artificial Larynx Speakers, dissertation. University of Kansas, Lawrence, 1975
7. Kalb MB: A Comparison of Esophageal Speech and Artificial Larynx Speech on the Basis of Intelligibility, thesis. University of Kansas, Lawrence, 1977

William R. Berry, Ph.D.

5.
Attitudes of Speech Pathologists and Otolaryngologists About Artificial Larynges

Before I review information related to the attitudes of our colleagues in medicine and speech pathology, it will be productive for you to examine your own opinions concerning the use of artificial larynx devices for alaryngeal speech. Using the scale from Table 5-1, rate your reactions to the ten statements in Table 5-2 in the *Before* column. Later, either after reading this chapter or the remainder of the book, re-rate yourself in the *After* column to determine whether you have changed your opinions. It is important that you complete this exercise now so that you will not be biased by any of the material to be presented. So go ahead; play a little solitaire on Table 5-2.

After completing the short exercise, compare your opinions with the average ratings of the ten statements in Table 5-3 from a group of 35 otolaryngologists (Column A), and then with those of 25 speech pathologists (Columns D and E). Both groups were asked to respond to the ten attitude statements using the rating scale in Table 5-1. Their average ratings, as well as the standard deviations for each statement, are summarized in Table 5-3.

For those clinicians who may not have much background in statistics, the standard deviation (SD) equals zero (0.00) if there is perfect agreement among all group members on any one statement. This actually occurred when the seven physicians in Hospital I (Column B) rated statement (3) with a -3, statistically resulting in a mean $(\bar{x})$ value of -3.00 and a 0.00 standard deviation. Such a rating is unusual; an SD almost always reflects some disagreement (i.e., will be greater than zero). Logically there is higher agreement among judges when the SD is lower, and vice versa. Assuming statistically a normal distribution of ratings, 95 percent of the ratings will fall

Table 5-1.
Scale Utilized for Rating Exercise (Table 5-2)
and Attitude Survey (Table 5-3).

Scale Value	Description
+3	Strongly agree
+2	Agree
+1	Agree with minor exceptions or reservations
0	Neutral; don't know; or not enough information or experience to respond intelligently
−1	Disagree with minor exceptions or reservations
−2	Disagree
−3	Strongly disagree

within ±2 SD. For example, if a group mean rating is −1.00 with an SD of 1.00, 95 percent of the ratings (or ± SD) fall between scale points −3 and +1. As the SD gets smaller, the group agreement increases. Thus, if the SD is 0.50 with a mean of −1.00, 95 percent of the ratings fall between −2 and 0.

ATTITUDES OF OTOLARYNGOLOGISTS

Let us consider the attitudes of otolaryngologists, whose life-saving surgery creates the aphonic condition the laryngectomee must face and conquer to speak again. In most instances patients place a tremendous amount of trust in their physicians. Therefore the surgeon can have a powerful, persuasive affect on the patient as he explains the effects of the surgery. If the surgeon expresses a bias for one type of speech rehabilitation, it is likely that the patient's attitudes will be significantly influenced. Because of this factor, it may be helpful to review the collective opinions of a group of surgeons (n = 35) concerning their views about artificial larynx devices. The ten statements from Table 5-2 were sent to 165 otolaryngologists and residents in eleven VA Hospitals. They used the rating scale presented in Table 5-1 and responded anonymously. Only 35 surgeons (21 percent) returned the questionnaires! The data are summarized in Columns A, B, and C of Table 5-3.

The mean and standard deviation for each of the ten statements from the total group of physicians are presented in Column A. Columns B and C summarize the opinions of physicians from two of the eleven hospitals sampled. They were the only two hospitals from which the number of surveys returned by physicians (Column B = 7 and Column C = 9) was great enough to make such a comparison.

Table 5-2.
Rating Exercise. Rate Each Statement Using Table 5-1.

Attitude Statement	Before	After
1. Hospital personnel often bias patients in favor of esophageal speech.		
2. Esophageal speech sounds better than artificial larynx speech, regardless of the level of intelligibility.		
3. An artificial larynx should not be issued to a patient until he or she has had an adequate opportunity to initiate esophageal sound.		
4. The laryngectomee should be given the opportunity to choose the type of speech developed after surgery.		
5. Being responsible for the patient's medical well-being, the surgeon should decide the type of alaryngeal communication (esophageal speech vs. artificial aid) that is most appropriate and so counsel the patient.		
6. Artificial laryngeal aids should be issued to the patients as soon as possible after surgery.		
7. Positive and negative factors concerning both artificial larynx speech and esophageal speech should be fully explained to a laryngectomized patient as soon as possible after surgery.		
8. The speech pathologist should decide the type of alaryngeal communication (esophageal speech vs. artificial larynx speech) that is most appropriate and so counsel the patient.		
9. An artificial larynx should not be used during esophageal speech therapy because it will significantly impede the progress of the latter.		
10. Most artificial larynx speakers are easier to understand (based upon your experience) over the telephone than most esophageal speakers.		

By reviewing the data in Column A, two points become apparent: the average ratings are relatively close to 0.00 on most of the statements; and the standard deviations are quite high. In general, these figures indicate that the surgeons expressed a wide variety of opinions, and that the group opinion tended toward the center of the scale. There was a moderate reflection of group agreement ($\bar{x} = 1.80$) on statement (7), indicating that the group favored presenting positive and negative information to patients concerning both esophageal and artificial larynx speech. However, an SD of 1.60

Table 5-3.
Data Summarizing Average Ratings ($\bar{x}$) and Standard Deviations (SD) for Five Groups.

Statement No. (Table 5-2)	A	B	C	D	E
1	$\bar{x}$ = 0.71 SD = 1.54	$\bar{x}$ = 1.57 SD = 1.13	$\bar{x}$ = 0.67 SD = 1.50	$\bar{x}$ = 0.96 SD = 1.90	$\bar{x}$ = 2.25* SD = 0.79
2	$\bar{x}$ = 0.61 SD = 1.93	$\bar{x}$ = 0.43 SD = 2.44	$\bar{x}$ = 0.50 SD = 1.59	$\bar{x}$ = −1.71 SD = 1.65	$\bar{x}$ = 2.54* SD = 0.59
3	$\bar{x}$ = −0.06 SD = 2.30	$\bar{x}$ = −3.00 SD = 0.00	$\bar{x}$ = 1.56 SD = 1.13	$\bar{x}$ = −2.46 SD = 0.72	$\bar{x}$ = −2.67 SD = 0.56
4	$\bar{x}$ = 1.14 SD = 1.40	$\bar{x}$ = 1.71 SD = 0.76	$\bar{x}$ = 0.44 SD = 1.59	$\bar{x}$ = 1.83 SD = 1.17	$\bar{x}$ = 2.42* SD = 0.78
5	$\bar{x}$ = −0.31 SD = 1.59	$\bar{x}$ = −0.85 SD = 1.68	$\bar{x}$ = −0.11 SD = 1.05	$\bar{x}$ = −2.75 SD = 0.44	$\bar{x}$ = −2.83 SD = 0.38
6	$\bar{x}$ = 1.11 SD = 1.56	$\bar{x}$ = 2.57 SD = 0.53	$\bar{x}$ = 0.33 SD = 1.66	$\bar{x}$ = 2.04 SD = 0.91	$\bar{x}$ = 2.25 SD = 0.74
7	$\bar{x}$ = 1.80 SD = 1.60	$\bar{x}$ = 2.43 SD = 0.79	$\bar{x}$ = 1.00 SD = 1.94	$\bar{x}$ = 1.67 SD = 1.69	$\bar{x}$ = 2.54* SD = 0.66
8	$\bar{x}$ = 0.26 SD = 1.70	$\bar{x}$ = 0.43 SD = 1.90	$\bar{x}$ = 0.33 SD = 1.32	$\bar{x}$ = 0.12 SD = 1.96	$\bar{x}$ = −1.71* SD = 1.23
9	$\bar{x}$ = −0.03 SD = 1.65	$\bar{x}$ = −1.81 SD = 1.21	$\bar{x}$ = 0.33 SD = 1.50	$\bar{x}$ = −1.83 SD = 1.40	$\bar{x}$ = −2.62* SD = 0.50
10	$\bar{x}$ = −0.09 SD = 1.09	$\bar{x}$ = −0.14 SD = 0.90	$\bar{x}$ = 0.00 SD = 1.12	$\bar{x}$ = 0.54 SD = 1.61	$\bar{x}$ = 0.92 SD = 1.53

(A) 35 surgeons, (B) 7 surgeons in Hospital I, (C) 9 surgeons in Hospital II, (D) 25 speech pathologists before training conference, (E) same 25 speech pathologists after training conference.

* Indicates significant difference between means in Columns D and E at .05 level; that is, the mean score for the post-conference survey statement is significantly different from the pre-conference mean rating.

indicates that a number of physicians were undecided or disagreed with the statement.

Slight agreement by the group was also registered on statements (4) and (6). The SDs were high enough, however, to make questionable any interpretation regarding the surgeons' belief that it is the patient's right to choose the type of communication he prefers, and that an artificial larynx should be issued to a laryngectomee immediately after surgery. The surgeons as a group actually seemed to have trouble agreeing on any of the issues.

In Columns B and C the data for two of the eleven hospitals are presented. The data from Hospital I (Column B) reflects opinions with a significant amount of agreement on several statements. Conversely, the data from Hospital II (Column C) does not exhibit agreement. Since the size of these two groups is small, it is unfair to assume that either set of data reflects a true attitude of surgeons. However, it is worth noting that the surgeons in Hospital I polarized their opinions enough to rate statement (3) exactly the same (-3). This agreement indicates displeasure with the idea that artificial aids should not be issued until esophageal sound is achieved. Apparently tradition, procedure, or communication has influenced this group of physicians so that early issuance of an artificial larynx is not perceived as an impedance to the acquisition of esophageal voice. But the data from Hospital II indicates that the surgeons disagreed concerning this issue. Relatively high agreement also was expressed by the surgeons in Hospital I for statements (4), (6), and (7). Conversely the surgeons in Hospital II did not agree, exhibiting instead a wide diversity of opinion.

We may speculate that the factors which cause such variance of opinion among the surgeons from the two hospitals are:

1. Clinical procedures relative to the timing of issuing artificial larynx devices.
2. Actual and/or perceived percentage of patients who develop esophageal speech.
3. Amount of training.
4. Exposure to artificial larynx devices.
5. Rapport between ENT and speech pathology services.

ATTITUDES OF SPEECH PATHOLOGISTS

In January 1976 I coordinated a conference sponsored by the VA Southeastern Regional Medical Education Center in Birmingham, Alabama. A number of speech-language pathologists working for the VA hospital system in the southeastern region of the United States were invited to attend this conference.[1] When planning the conference and discussing the use of artificial larynges with a number of colleagues experienced in working with laryngectomized patients, I realized that this conference might be one of the first, if not the first, conference devoted to the topic of artificial larynx devices. In contrast many courses, workshops, and conferences have been offered that relate to esophageal speech.

This fact alone illustrates the bias in favor of esophageal speech. At the Birmingham conference, speech clinicians reported that their university clinical training in the use of alaryngeal devices had been inadequate. Most indicated that they were shown a few types of artificial larynges, but that

Shirley J. Salmon, Ph.D.

6.
Patients Talk Back

The two preceding chapters by Goldstein and by Berry emphasize that despite inconclusive information concerning listener preferences, groups of speech pathologists or otolaryngologists exhibit ambivalent attitudes concerning artificial larynges. Thus it seems reasonable to assume that some professionals working with laryngectomees are aware that they communicate such ambivalence to patients. To compensate for their negative viewpoints, and to offer some encouragement, the positive aspects of esophageal speech are frequently overemphasized.

Other professionals seem to feel totally justified in their negativism concerning artificial larynges. They are quick to discourage use of the devices and seem to feel confident when defending such a position.

From professionals in either category, laryngectomized patients are likely to interpret that esophageal speech is the preferred if not the only method of alaryngeal speech. Think for a moment about how such an idea may be communicated. Either pre- or postoperatively, isn't esophageal speech stressed by the surgeon, the nurse, the laryngectomee visitor, and speech pathologist? Aren't most of the booklets and pamphlets we distribute geared toward explanations of esophageal speech? Think about the American Cancer Society's film shown so frequently at bedside, "You Will Speak Again." Speak how? With esophageal speech, of course.

Consider the meetings of New Voice Clubs throughout the country. If 40 percent of the laryngectomized population does not communicate by esophageal speech, it is reasonable to expect that 40 percent of the New Voice Club membership will use artificial larynx devices. This type of representation does not exist in any of the clubs with which I am familiar.

Could it be that artificial larynx speakers feel unwelcome or like second-class citizens when they attend such club meetings? When thinking about the meetings I've attended, I realize that there have been many talks about esophageal speech and many sessions devoted to esophageal speech instruction. However, I doubt that many meetings have provided information about use of artificial larynx devices or have provided instruction for their use.

Further, most graduate classes, seminars, or workshops fail to provide lessons about teaching proficient communication with artificial larynx devices. Only since 1975 have lessons for artificial larynx speakers been provided at the annual convention of the International Association for Laryngectomees (IAL). And 1976 was the first year that the board of directors agreed to provide funds to purchase and maintain a supply of various types of artificial larynx devices for demonstration at future IAL conventions.

These are only some of the ways in which we have communicated the idea that esophageal speech is the only method of speech following laryngectomy. As we've been "selling" esophageal speech, the communication proficiency of speakers who use artificial devices essentially has been ignored.

As a means of checking the accuracy of these ideas, I conducted a questionnaire study of artificial larynx speakers in 1976. (See Appendix, pp. 50–53.) Some of the information obtained from that study is presented here. Perhaps it will help us appreciate the type of experiences that many laryngectomized patients are having with instructors of alaryngeal speech.

SURVEY REPORT

Respondents

Responses were obtained from 50 of the 65 artificial larynx speakers to whom questionnaires were mailed; that is, 76 percent responded, which is a high rate of return. To avoid bias due to geographic location, ten speech pathologists living in various parts of the country were asked to provide the names of at least five artificial larynx speakers who would be willing to complete the rather lengthy questionnaire forms. Responses subsequently came from people living in New York, Pennsylvania, Ohio, Mississippi, Iowa, Florida, Texas, California, Kansas, Missouri, Minnesota, and Arkansas.

The ages of the speakers ranged from 34 to 77, with a mean age of 58.45 years at the time they underwent laryngectomy. They were between the ages of 45 and 79 with a mean age of 63.87 years at the time they completed the questionnaire forms. On the average they had been using their artificial larynx devices about 5.42 years. Six respondents were females and 44 were males.

Visitations

Twenty-five of the 50 respondents (50 percent) received preoperative visits from speech pathologists and esophageal speakers or artificial larynx speakers; 42 of the 50 (84 percent) received postoperative visits from one or more of these persons. Six of the 50 (12 percent) received neither pre- nor postoperative visits from a speech pathologist, an esophageal speaker, or an artificial larynx speaker. There was a total of 292 pre- and postoperative visits with 142 (48 percent) made by speech pathologist, 98 (34 percent) made by esophageal speakers, and 52 (18 percent) made by artificial larynx speakers. This tally regarding visits from esophageal speakers and artificial larynx speakers supports one reported by Goldstein.[1] It indicates that newly laryngectomized patients receive alaryngeal speech demonstrations that are biased in favor of esophageal speech.

Introduction to Artificial Larynx Devices

Slightly fewer than two-thirds of the group (60 percent), were introduced to an artificial larynx by a speech pathologist. Eleven (22 percent) were first given information about an artificial larynx by another laryngectomee and nine (18 percent) were told about it by other persons—a surgeon, two American Cancer Society representatives, a son who was an electrical engineer for Western Electric, a mother-in-law, a friend, and three salesmen.

Of the 40 speakers (80 percent) who received instructions about use of the artificial larynx, 32 (80 percent) were from a speech pathologist and five (13 percent) were from another laryngectomee. One received instructions from both a speech pathologist and a laryngectomee, one from a graduate student, and one from a salesman who sold one type of artificial larynx device.

Introduction to Esophageal Speech

The percentages are somewhat different for those patients who received instructions about esophageal speech. Thirty-seven (88 percent) of the 42 (84 percent) who reported receiving instructions about esophageal speech received them from a speech pathologist. Two received them from a laryngectomee, two received them from both a laryngectomee and a speech pathologist, and one received them from a graduate student. Thus, speech pathologists provided artificial larynx instruction to 80 percent and esophageal speech instruction to 88 percent of the patients studied. Keep these figures in mind.

The average amount of esophageal speech instruction for this group was 22 hours; six persons reported vague responses such as "many half-hour sessions" or "up to ten months of therapy sessions." Conversely the average amount of instruction for use of the artificial larynx was 2 hours. These findings support those of Goldstein[1]; the average length of instruction reported by his alaryngeal speech group was 18 hours for esophageal speech, and 2 hours for artificial larynx speech.

Types of Devices

The Western Electric No. 5 device was shown to 45 of the 50 artificial larynx speakers. Ten also were shown a Servox, five an Aurex, four a Cooper-Rand, one a Kett, one a Tokyo, and one an Osaka. When asked why they chose the artificial larynx they were using, some speakers checked more than one of the choices they were offered. (The choices overlapped so that it was difficult to convert the responses into percentages.) Some of the speakers indicated that they chose their particular model device because it was the only one they knew about; others indicated that it was because of availability, economy, or because it worked better for them than the others they had tried to use. The largest number of subjects, 30 (64 percent), indicated that someone they trusted had recommended it. Twenty-four (80 percent) indicated that the person they had trusted was a speech pathologist. In other instances it was a laryngectomee, a physician, or someone else.

Emotional Reactions to Use of Devices

Significantly, 43 (86 percent) speakers indicated that they did not feel apologetic or embarrassed about choosing to use an artificial larynx instead of esophageal speech. Even more significant were their answers to the next question, which was "If you felt apologetic or embarrassed, was it with speech pathologists, esophageal speakers, artificial larynx speakers, spouse/family members, surgeons, or others (specify)?" Although only seven speakers had previously indicated feelings of apology or embarrassment about choosing to use the artificial larynx, 16 (32 percent) indicated embarrassment with certain persons. Thirteen of the 16 reported that they felt apologetic or embarrassed with surgeons, eight with speech pathologists, nine with esophageal speakers, eight with friends or spouse/family members, four with artificial larynx speakers, and one with customers.

Instructions for Use of Devices

One of the most interesting findings from this survey came from answers to the next question, "Please check the information you were given about the type of artificial larynx you are now using." Thirteen choices were provided:

- a. Purchase price.
- b. Maintenance cost, i.e. batteries, replacement parts, repair.
- c. Where to purchase batteries.
- d. Where to send device for repair.
- e. How to turn it on and off.
- f. Proper placement, i.e. on the neck, over the stoma, in the mouth.
- g. Synchronizing sound with lip and tongue movements.
- h. Need for clear pronunciation of sounds and words.
- i. How to vary pitch to improve the meaning of your message.
- j. How to vary loudness to improve the meaning of your message.
- k. How to vary loudness so it is appropriate for the occasion.
- l. How to make the speech sound more rhythmical.
- m. How to blend words together or cut them short to improve the meaning of the message.

In looking over this list, remember that of the 40 speakers in this group who received instruction about use of the artificial larynx, five received them from a laryngectomee, 32 from both a speech pathologist and a laryngectomee, one from a graduate student, and one from a salesman. Apparently the nine speakers who received no instructions taught themselves. Also remember that the average amount of instruction received was only two hours.

Of this group of patients, 31 (62 percent) received information about the purchase price; 27 (54 percent) were told about maintenance costs; 27 (54 percent) were advised where to purchase batteries; and 35 (70 percent) were told where to send their device for repair. The information provided most often, but not always, was that concerning items (e) and (f). Forty patients (80 percent) were instructed in turning the device on and off, and 35 (70 percent) were advised about the need for proper placement. From this point most of the percentages become distressingly smaller; fewer than half of the group reported that they had received information about the remaining items (g) through (m). Twenty-two (47 percent) of the speakers were encouraged to synchronize sound with articulatory movements; 22 (47 percent) were told of the need for precise articulation; and 19 (40 percent) were taught how to vary their pitch. Only 16 (34 percent) were taught how to vary loudness for improving the meaning of their message, and how to make the volume appropriate for different occasions. A slightly larger number, 18 (38 percent), were encouraged to make their speech sound more rhythmical. Finally, 19 (40 percent) were instructed about the advantages of phrasing.

SUMMARY

These percentages indicate that speech pathologists teach the mechanical aspects of using an artificial larynx but not the refinement techniques. This finding is reminiscent of an article written by Knepflar,[2] in which he suggested that too many esophageal speakers are dismissed from esophageal speech treatment before being introduced to concepts and drills that emphasize pitch, volume, and phrasing. He encouraged using these techniques to refine esophageal speech. Many of us heeded his advice. Now we need to adopt his idea of refinement and apply it to artificial larynx speech.

Knox and Anneberg[3] provided evidence to support the idea that instructions about the use of artificial larynx devices can be beneficial. They investigated the effect of different signal-to-noise ratios on the comprehension of electronic larynx speech. One of their conclusions is particularly relevant. They stated that appropriate placement of an electronic artificial larynx can create a 4 dB difference between the unmodulated tone of the instrument and the voice signal. Such a difference allows listeners to demonstrate a high degree of comprehension. If instructions about proper placement increase listener comprehension, imagine what effect might be gained from instructions regarding other aspects of artificial larynx usage!

To those clinicians who continue to feel leery about artificial larynx devices, let me stress the fact that 40 percent of laryngectomized patients do not acquire esophageal speech. And some of those who do use esophageal speech have such limited skills that they may communicate more easily and effectively with artificial larynges. These two different groups of laryngectomees may feel less apologetic about using artificial larynx devices and use them more effectively if we:

1. Arrange for more postoperative demonstrations of artificial larynx speech.
2. Spend more time providing instructions about use of the devices.
3. Improve the quality of our instructions so that we do not just teach the mechanical aspects of the artificial larynx, but in addition teach the refinements of artificial larynx speech.
4. Develop criteria for both the evaluation of proficiency with the artificial larynx and dismissal from artificial larynx speech therapy.

CONCLUSION

Currently we are encouraging negative attitudes about the use and possible effectiveness of the artificial larynx by sending artificial larynx speakers into the *speaking* world without the communication skills we are supposed to know and care about most. This results in a self-fulfilling prophecy: we say the devices are bad, and we introduce them late in the therapy program and without proper instruction. Then we nod our heads knowingly when patients use them poorly and imply that we "knew it all the time"; the devices are unsatisfactory.

The data cited in this chapter indicate that speech pathologists frequently fail to provide adequate instructions in the use of artificial larynx devices. We need to begin providing quality treatment by changing our techniques for the patients' sake.

REFERENCES

1. Goldstein L: A Study of the Relationship Between Adience–Abience Scores and Judgments of Verbal Communication Proficiency of a Group of Esophageal Speakers and a Group of Artificial Larynx Speakers, dissertation. University of Kansas, Lawrence, 1974
2. Knepflar K: Therapy approaches for the improvement and refinement of pseudovoice in laryngectomized speakers. NZ Speech Ther. 18:18–22, 1963
3. Knox A, Anneberg M: The effects of training in comprehension of electrolaryngeal speech. J Commun Disorders 6:110–120, 1973

Appendix

QUESTIONNAIRE FOR ARTIFICIAL LARYNX SPEAKERS

1. Name _____ 2. Sex _____ Male _____ Female

3. Address _____

4. Birthdate _____ 5. Age at time of laryngectomy _____

6. Before surgery how many visits did you receive from:

    a. a speech pathologist _____
    b. a laryngectomee using esophageal speech _____
    c. a laryngectomee using an artificial larynx _____

7. After surgery how many visits did you receive from:

    a. a speech pathologist _____
    b. a laryngectomee using esophageal speech _____
    c. a laryngectomee using an artificial larynx _____

8. The first person who introduced you to the artificial larynx was:

    a. a speech pathologist _____
    b. another laryngectomee _____
    c. a salesman from a company that manufactures one type of device _____
    d. surgeon _____
    e. other (specify) _____

9. How many half-hours of instruction did you receive for:

    a. esophageal speech _____ half-hours
    b. artificial larynx speech _____ half-hours

10. If you did not receive any instruction for esophageal speech, would you like to have had it available?

    Yes _____   No _____

11. If you did not receive any instruction in the use of an artificial larynx, would you like to have had it available?

    Yes _____ No _____

12. If you did receive instruction, by whom was it offered?

    Artificial larynx instruction

    a. speech pathologist _____
    b. laryngectomee _____
    c. doctor _____
    d. other _____

    Esophageal speech instruction

    a. speech pathologist _____
    b. laryngectomee _____
    c. doctor _____
    d. other _____

13. Did you feel that you could choose to use an artificial larynx instead of esophageal speech without being apologetic or embarrassed?

    Yes _____ No _____

14. If you felt apologetic or embarrassed, was it with:

    a. speech pathologists   _____ Yes _____ No
    b. esophageal speakers   _____ Yes _____ No
    c. artificial larynx speakers _____ Yes _____ No
    d. spouse or family members   _____ Yes _____ No
    e. surgeons   _____ Yes _____ No
    f. other (specify)   _____ Yes _____ No

15. About which artificial larynx devices did you receive information?

    a. Bell Telephone Battery Operated _____
    b. Aurex "Neovox" _____
    c. Servox Speech Aid _____
    d. Cooper-Rand _____
    e. Yamamura Artificial Larynx _____
    f. Tokyo Artificial Larynx _____
    g. Other (specify) _____

16. What *one* reason was the most important one for choosing the artificial larynx you are now using?

    a. The only one you knew about _____
    b. The one most readily available _____
    c. The most economical _____
    d. The one recommended by someone you trusted:
       (1) doctor _____   (3) speech pathologist _____
       (2) laryngectomee _____ (4) other (specify) _____

17. Please check the information you were given about the type of artificial larynx you are now using.
    a. Purchase price _____
    b. Maintenance cost—batteries, replacement parts, repair _____
    c. Where to purchase batteries _____
    d. Where to send the device for repair _____
    e. How to turn it off and on _____
    f. Proper placement (on the neck, over the stoma, in the mouth) _____
    g. Synchronizing sound with lip and tongue movements _____
    h. Need for clear pronunciation of sounds and words _____
    i. How to vary pitch to improve the meaning of your message _____
    j. How to vary loudness so that it helps the meaning of your message _____
    k. How to vary loudness so that it is appropriate for the occasion _____
    l. How to make your speech sound more rhythmical _____
    m. How to blend words together or cut them short to improve the meaning of your message _____

18. Have you ever attended a local New Voice Club meeting?

    Yes _____   No _____

19. Do you attend at least half of the local New Voice Club meetings?

    Yes _____   No _____

20. If you do attend the meetings, what do you like about them?
    a. Opportunity to socialize with other laryngectomees _____
    b. Opportunity to share information and common problems _____
    c. Opportunity to inspire or help others _____
    d. Provides a fun social activity that you need in your life _____
    e. Speech improvement classes _____
    f. Other (specify) _____

21. If you do not attend the meetings, why not?
    a. Transportation is too difficult _____
    b. Meeting time conflicts with other meeting commitments _____
    c. No desire to socialize with other laryngectomees _____
    d. No need for additional social activities _____
    e. Do not believe they want artificial larynx speakers to attend _____

  f. Were told not to use the artificial larynx and it made you angry _____
  g. Did not know there were such meetings _____
  h. No such clubs organized in this area _____
  i. Other (specify) _____

22. If there is additional information you believe I should have, please provide it here:

Section III

ARTIFICIAL LARYNX DEVICES

This section includes complete information concerning artificial larynx devices. A historical review provides a perspective of how today's artificial larynx devices were developed. The instructions, modifications, and adjustments for each instrument are given. Also included is a chapter describing the analysis of good and poor speech produced with an electronic artificial larynx. This information should enable the reader to make objective judgments about selecting and evaluating artificial larynx devices.

Eric D. Blom, Ph.D.

7.
The Artificial Larynx:
Past and Present

From early pioneering events—description of the physiological principle of esophageal phonation by Reynaud in 1841; the earliest published design for an artificial larynx by Czermak in 1859; Billroth's accomplishment of the first laryngectomy in 1873—stems a colorful history of laryngeal substitutes. It is a chronicle of the accomplishments that have paved the way for literally all artificial larynges available today.

The following pages provide (a) a review of the historical development of artificial larynges; (b) a comprehensive discussion of currently available manufactured artificial larynges and suggestions for their modification; and (c) a brief orientation to some combined surgical-prosthetic approaches to voice restoration being used in the United States. This chapter is intended as a major review of prosthetic methods of alaryngeal voice restoration, but I recognize that the information is not all-inclusive.

HISTORICAL DEVELOPMENT

The historical development of the artificial larynx has been described well by Kallen,[1] Lebrun,[2] Arnold,[3] and Hanson.[4] Prosthetic larynges frequently have been categorized according to either the nature of the power source used to activate artificial sound production, or the anatomical point at which the sound source is introduced into the human vocal tract. In this chapter a combination of the two classification systems is utilized. The major delineations are pneumatic and electronic, with electronic devices subdivided into mouth-type and neck-type.

The pneumatic artificial larynx is powered by air from the tracheostoma which in turn activates vibratory response in a metal or plastic reed, rubber membrane, or human tissue. Electronic artificial larynges are basically battery-powered impulse generators that produce sound either by activating an electronic transducer or by driving a mechanical piston against a rigid membrane. The term "mouth-type" electronic larynges usually refers to electronic sound sources which either originate from within the mouth or are held up to the mouth. Terms synonymous in the literature with mouth-type include oral, intra-oral, and extra-oral. "Neck-type" devices introduce sound into the pharynx through the cervical soft tissue by applying the vibrator against the neck. Synonymous terms include transcervical and throat-type.

Pneumatic Artificial Larynx

Design of the first known artificial larynx is credited to a Czech physiologist named Johann Czermak,[2] who in 1859 created it for use by a tracheotomized eighteen-year-old girl suffering from complete laryngeal stenosis. The design of this remarkably advanced, external laryngeal prosthesis consisted of a small flexible metal reed housed in a tube leading from the tracheostoma to the mouth. Sound could be produced when the reed was activated by tracheal air flow. Although it is unclear whether this prototype pneumatic artificial larynx ever actually was constructed and used, Kallen[1] reports that Brucke assembled and successfully applied a pneumatic instrument presumably based on Czermak's design.

In 1873 Josef Leiter[2] made an internal pneumatic artificial larynx for the patient on whom the first known laryngectomy surgery was performed by Billroth. Leiter's instrument capitalized on the presence of a pharyngeal passage, leading to the mouth, that customarily remained following the laryngeal amputation advocated by Billroth.[3] Leiter's artificial larynx had three components: a laryngeal, tracheal, and phonatory cannula. The curved tracheal cannula was inserted through the tracheostoma and down into the trachea. The laryngeal cannula (containing the phonatory cannula and metal reed) was introduced upward into the pharyngeal passage. The opening to the laryngeal cannula was protected by a spring-loaded metal lid (trap door) designed to prevent fouling of the reed by aspiration of foreign matter during swallowing, and to function as an epiglottis. The user of the device breathed through the tracheal cannula. Voice could be produced by occluding the tracheal orifice and directing the expiratory airstream across the sound-producing reed in the upper portion of the prosthesis.

In 1874 Billroth's assistant, Carl Gussenbauer,[2] modified Leiter's artificial larynx by shortening the reed and making it more easily removable. He also incorporated a filter mechanism in the orifice of the tracheal cannula to more effectively prevent foreign matter from entering the prosthesis and fouling the reed mechanism.

Modifications to Leiter's principle of an internal pneumatic artificial larynx were offered in 1877 by Irvine and Fould, in 1881 by Bruns, and in 1893 by Wolff. Irvine and Fould redesigned the laryngeal cannula, which had been difficult to insert, so that it could be inserted into the pharyngeal passage before the tracheal cannula was inserted into the trachea. They also experimented with various reed materials and devised a reed that could easily be removed from the prosthesis for cleaning purposes. Bruns further improved the basic design by:

1. Replacing the rigid laryngeal cannula with a flexible cannula.
2. Providing a plug attached to a curved wire that could be inserted into the laryngeal cannula during eating to prevent leakage.
3. Replacing the metal reed with one made of a rubber material, which reportedly created a more natural voice.
4. Suggesting a one-way respiration valve in the opening to the tracheal cannula, presumably to obviate the need to occlude this opening with a finger during speech. Wolff suggested a few modifications to Bruns' prosthesis including a redesigned respiration valve that permitted greater pulmonary exchange, and a reed mechanism that could be shortened or lengthened to provide pitch variability.

Interest in internal pneumatic laryngeal substitutes was abandoned around the turn of the century with the acceptance of Gluck's[3] important modification to the surgical technique of laryngectomy. Gluck advocated attaching the tracheal stump to the skin of the neck and suturing the pharyngeal passage shut to prevent pulmonary aspiration of saliva and nutrients permanently. This modification terminated the point of entrance into the vocal tract which had been occupied previously by the reed mechanism.

In 1877 Carl Stork,[2] presumably inspired by Czermak's initial efforts, designed an external pneumatic artificial larynx. Although he originally designed it to be powered by air pressure from a hand-squeezed bulb, Stork later modified it to attach to the user's tracheal cannula. Pulmonary air issuing from the trachea activated a reed in the instrument, and the ensuing sound was directed to the mouth by an external piece of tubing.

In 1892 Hochenegg[2] duplicated Stork's external reed larynx driven by air-pump. His device consisted of a bellows that was strapped to the user's side and activated when the user pumped his arm. A tube conveyed air from the bellows to a reed positioned in a tube. The distal end of the tube was introduced into the vocal tract through the user's nose.

Gottstein[3] in 1899 also contributed to the refinement of the external pneumatic larynx. His device was comprised of a tracheal cannula with an inflatable rubber cuff, which insured an air-tight seal at the tracheostoma; a wire-reinforced rubber tube, which led to a small valved cylinder containing a reed; and a curved metal tube which could be inserted in the corner of the mouth. In the succeeding years 1899 to 1914, Gluck,[4] Martin,[2] Tapia,[4] and Onodi and Stockman[2] designed other innovative external pneumatic larynges.

In 1926 Western Electric marketed a pneumatic artificial larynx which reportedly was designed by MacKenty, Fletcher, and Lane.[2] It was known as the Western Electric No. 1 Type, and was comprised of a padded tracheal connector which could be strapped over the tracheostoma, a stretched rubber membrane housed in a small cylinder, and a short metal mouth-tube. The user breathed through a hole in the side of the small cylinder. By occluding this hole with a finger, tracheal air could be directed through the device to activate the rubber membrane and produce voice.

Elmer McKesson[5] filed a patent in 1927 for an artificial larynx called the Vocophone. This unique instrument consisted of dual, metal soundchambers, each housing a separate rubber membrane which could be adjusted in width, thickness, and length to produce various pitches. Simultaneous activation of the two differently tuned vibrators reportedly created a pitch blend which resulted in a more natural-sounding artificial voice.

In 1930 Western Electric introduced the No. 2 Type pneumatic artificial larynx. This instrument was designed by Reisz[6,7] and replaced the earlier No. 1 Type, which had turned out to be unsatisfactory because its membrane vibrator deteriorated rapidly and had to be replaced frequently.* The No. 2 Type was comprised of a flexible rubber tube which was attached to a soft, circular stoma cover at one end, and to a cylindrical chamber housing a noncorrosive metal reed at the other end (see Figure 7-1). Sound produced by the vibrating reed was transmitted to the mouth through another short tube. This artificial larynx was sold with a pre-set reed to produce a highpitched tone for female users (No. 2 BA) and a lower-pitched tone for male users (No. 2 AA). The No. 2 Type was a popular artificial larynx for 30 years, before being replaced by the Western Electric No. 5 electrolarynx in 1959.

Electronic Artificial Larynx

MOUTH-TYPE LARYNGES

The first electronic larynx, a mouth-type device, is reported to have been conceived by Gluck[3] in 1905. It consisted of a portable springoperated phonograph housed in a sound-isolated container. The source of

---

* G. Smith 1977: personal communication.

THE ARTIFICIAL LARYNX: PAST AND PRESENT

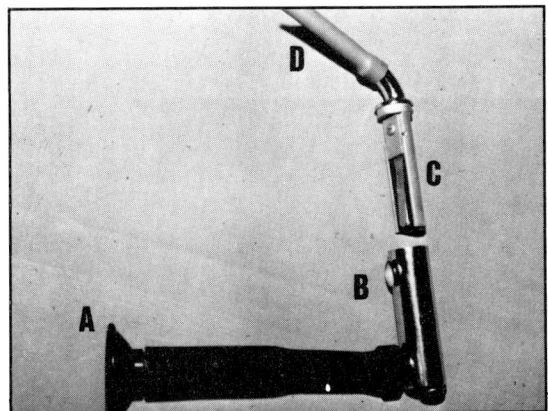

Figure 7-1. Western Electric artificial larynx No. 2 Type. A. Stoma cover. B. Reed chamber. C. Reed. D. Mouth tube.

sound for this ingenious artificial larynx was a sustained tone that had been produced by a singer and recorded on a disc. When the unit was activated, the prerecorded human vocal tone was transmitted via a tube to the user's mouth and articulated into speech.

In 1914 Gluck experimented with another mouth-type electronic larynx. This device was an electromagnetically-activated telephone receiver which could be concealed in a dental plate. The prerecorded tone of a singer, reproduced by a portable phonograph, energized the membrane of the receiver located in the mouth. The user had to be willing to tolerate a cord running from his mouth to the phonograph.

Pilcher[2] in 1957 developed a wireless induction system designed to transmit radio signals from a battery-powered pocket oscillator to a small receiver concealed in a denture. The oscillator was activated by a switch that was located in front of the tracheostoma and was sensitive to increases in expiratory air pressure. The user could activate the sound source in his mouth without using his hands and without having a wire leading out of his mouth. As far as can be determined, Pilcher's artificial larynx was never manufactured.

In 1957 Cooper and Millard[8,9] filed a patent for a mouth-type electronic artificial larynx. Cooper's device was comprised of a battery-pack carried in the pocket, an on–off switch located under the armpit, and a wire leading from the battery-pack to a diaphragm which was plugged into the lateral aspect of an upper dental plate. A slight squeeze of the arm produced a sound in the mouth that could be articulated into speech.

Tait and Tait[10] also developed a denture-mounted electronic larynx at about the same time as Cooper. The prototype of the Tait "Oral Vibrator" was an electromagnetic diaphragm concealed in the center of an upper dental plate. A wire led out of the corner of the user's mouth to a small box containing a battery-powered, transistorized audio-oscillator. When a switch on the box was pressed, the electromagnetic diaphragm was activated to produce sound. According to Lebrun,[2] Tait described a second prototype that improved on the first by eliminating the manually activated switch, battery-pack, and wire leading from the mouth. Rather, the oscillator, battery, and diaphragm were miniaturized and concealed in a dental plate. On–off activation of the unit was accomplished by pressure exerted with the tongue against specific locations on the prosthesis. The batteries could be re-energized by plugging a battery charger into the side of the unit at night, when the dental plate was not being worn.

The Danapipe is an additional mouth-type electronic larynx that warrants mention. This prosthesis, no longer available, was produced by Danavox International in Denmark.[2] It was comprised of miniaturized circuitry, a transducer, and a battery concealed in the bowl portion of a tobacco pipe. A switch on the side of the bowl activated the sound, which then was transmitted through the stem of the pipe to the user's mouth.

NECK-TYPE LARYNGES

Wright is credited with inventing the first neck-type electronic larynx in 1942.[11] Called the Sonovox, this instrument was comprised of a battery-powered oscillator housed in a cylindrical plastic case. The oscillator produced sound by driving a small piston at high velocity against a rigid membrane. The device was hand-held. Its power supply, which was connected by a cord to the handle, could be carried in the pocket or on a shoulder strap. Wright's artificial larynx was eventually produced by the Aurex Corporation of Chicago, Illinois—first as the Wright Electrolarynx, and currently as the Aurex Neovox M-520T. His design also inspired a similar electronic larynx known as the Kett Mark III, which was manufactured by the Kett Engineering Corporation of Santa Monica, California until being discontinued in 1970.

CURRENTLY AVAILABLE ARTIFICIAL LARYNGES

This section provides a review of currently available artificial larynges. In some instances home-made modifications are provided that, based on subjective clinical evaluation, might improve the design and versatility of a number of the instruments described. Pneumatic instruments are discussed first, followed by mouth-type and neck-type electronic larynges. Speech pathologists who intend to offer comprehensive alaryngeal speech therapy should be completely familiar with these instruments, be able to demonstrate their use either personally or with videotaped samples, and have available as many of them as possible for trial purposes.

Pneumatic Artificial Larynges

TOKYO ARTIFICIAL LARYNX

The Tokyo device is an inexpensive, Japanese-made instrument consisting of either a steel or soft rubber cover which fits over the stoma, a steel pipe leading to and away from a cylindrical chamber which houses a stretched rubber membrane held in position by a rubber band, and a plastic or rubber mouth-tube (Figures 7-2 and 7-3). The pitch can be varied by adjusting the width and tension of the vibrating membrane, or by varying breath pressure during use. Varying breath pressure also results in a significant variation in loudness. Speech with the Tokyo has been described by Weinberg and Riekena.[12]

Simple modifications to the Tokyo make it more functional. To negate the necessity of moving the Tokyo from the stoma on each inhalation, a $\frac{3}{8}$-inch hole drilled in the cylindrical body of the instrument provides a convenient finger-controlled breathing port (see Figure 7-4). A soft-flanged fistula tube serves nicely in cases where the standard steel or rubber tracheostoma cover doesn't adequately fit over the stoma. In rare instances when the user must wear a tracheal cannula, it may be necessary to replace the standard tracheostoma cover with a tapered suction-drainage tube which will fit into the cannula and provide an air-tight seal.

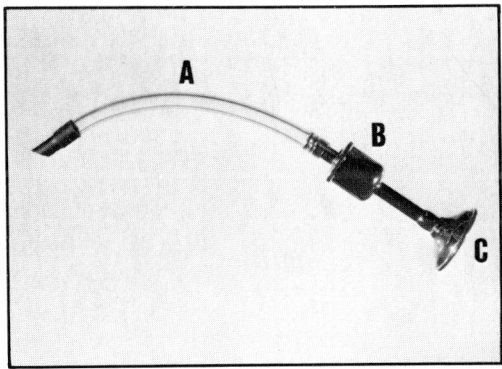

Figure 7-2. Tokyo artificial larynx. *A.* Mouth tube. *B.* Vibrator chamber. *C.* Steel stoma cover.

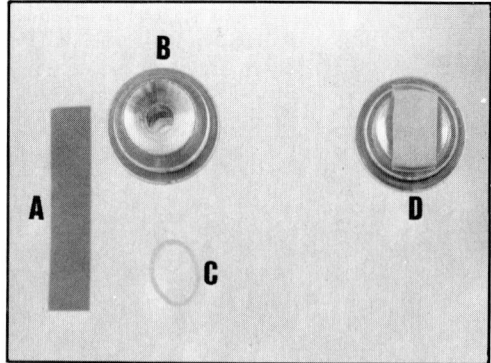

Figure 7-3. Tokyo artificial larynx vibrator assembly. A. Rubber membrane. B. Top view of chamber interior. C. Othodontic rubber band. D. Assembled vibrator.

Another effective modification with the Tokyo as well as with other mouth-type devices consists of using a dental saliva-ejector tube to replace the more conventional tygon mouth tubing (Figure 7-4). This type of tube offers the following advantages.

1. A wire running through the tubing gives firmness and at the same time makes it possible to bend the tubing into permanent shapes.
2. Greater thickness decreases sound radiation through the tubing wall.
3. A small, slitted cap over the end of the tube decreases intake of saliva and skin tissue into the tube orifice when the tube is in the mouth.

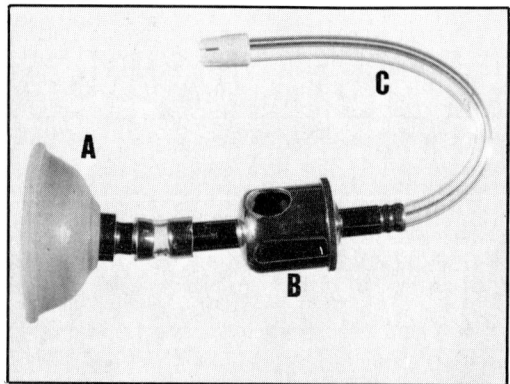

Figure 7-4. Modified Tokyo artificial larynx. A. Rubber stoma cover. B. Finger-controlled breathing port. C. Dental saliva-ejector tube.

The Tokyo is available from Mr. Red Woodward, 3132 Waits Avenue, Ft. Worth, Texas 76109, at an approximate cost of $25.00.

In 1975 Nelson, Parkin, and Pottor[13] described two modifications to the Tokyo. Rigidity and curvature of the mouth tube are achieved by constructing the tube out of pre-bent stainless steel and by capping the portion that actually goes into the mouth with a short piece of plastic tubing. To overcome the difficulties presented by an irregularly angled stoma, a swivel-joint connector is incorporated on the proximal end of the device, between the steel connecting tube and the tracheostoma cover. Information regarding purchase of this modified Tokyo is available from James L. Parkin, M.D., University of Utah College of Medicine, 50 N. Medical Drive, Salt Lake City, Utah 48132. Cost of the modified device is reported to be in excess of $140.00.

OSAKA ARTIFICIAL LARYNX

The Osaka artificial larynx is another Japanese-manufactured instrument and is basically similar to the Tokyo (Figure 7-5). The tracheostoma cover and housing for the rubber vibrator are made of lightweight plastic. It

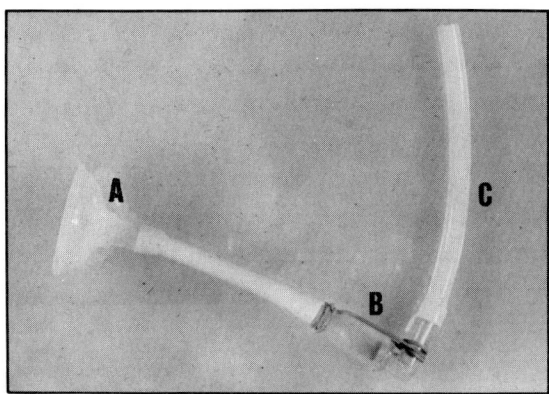

Figure 7-5. Osaka (Yamamura) artificial larynx. A. Stoma cover. B. Vibratory mechanism. C. Mouth tube.

is possible to change the pitch and loudness of the tone by altering the physical characteristics of the vibrator or by varying breath pressure during use. The Osaka is referred to by some as the Yamamura and it was formerly distributed by the late Reverend Yoshimi Yamamura.* The Osaka can be purchased from Mr. Red Woodward, 3132 Waits Avenue, Ft. Worth, Texas 76109 for approximately $25.00.

* R. Woodward 1976: personal communication.

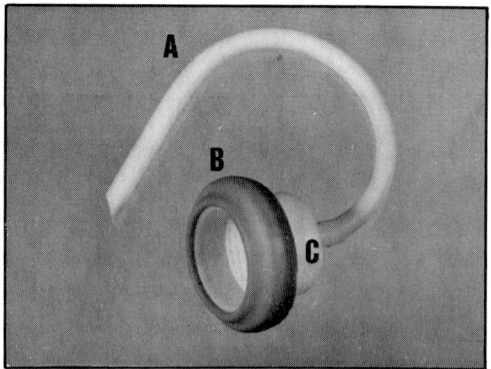

Figure 7-6. Van Humen (DSP8) artificial larynx. *A.* Mouth tube. *B.* Vibratory mechanism. *C.* Air-filled stoma cover.

VAN HUMEN ARTIFICIAL LARYNX ("DUTCH" DSP8)

The Van Humen artificial larynx has a plastic mouth-tube, nylon vibrator housing, adjustable rubber membrane, and an air-filled cover which fits over the stoma (Figure 7-6). The design permits the user to breathe normally and also to speak without removing the device from the stoma. This Dutch-made instrument is infrequently seen in the United States, but is available from Memacon, Pres. Kennedy Laan 263, P.O. Box 56, Velp 6200, Netherlands, at a cost of approximately $85.00.

NEHER 5000 ARTIFICIAL LARYNX

The Neher is a high quality polished chrome instrument basically consisting of a tracheostoma cover, a reed housing with a finger-control breathing port, a hard plastic reed, and a flexible clear plastic mouth-tube (Figure 7-7). The Neher is also available with a special tapered steel adaptor designed as an interconnector for use with a tracheal cannula. Physical properties of the reed can be altered (length, width, shape) to vary pitch characteristics and ease of tone initiation. This instrument can be purchased from the Neher Artificial Larynx Company, 103 6th Street, S.W., Kasson, Minnesota 55944, for approximately $70.00.

Electronic Mouth-Type Artificial Larynges

COOPER-RAND ELECTRONIC SPEECH AID

Probably the most widely known mouth-type electronic larynx is the Cooper-Rand. This instrument basically consists of a battery-powered pulse

THE ARTIFICIAL LARYNX: PAST AND PRESENT   67

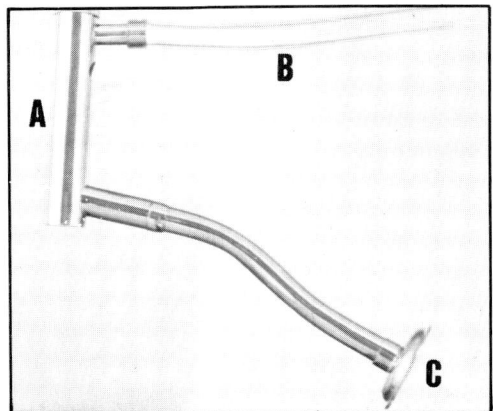

Figure 7-7. Neher 5000 artificial larynx. A. Reed chamber. B. Mouth tube. C. Stoma cover.

generator which connects by a wire to a hand-held tone generator (Figure 7-8). Sound is directed into the mouth by a short piece of plastic tubing. Switches incorporated on the instrument permit variation in both pitch and loudness. Recently the manufacturer of the Cooper-Rand made several needed improvements. The cords supplied with the instrument are now of a heavier gauge and thus are less likely to break. Both the conventional plastic mouth-tubes and the saliva-ejector tubes described previously are included with the instrument. The manufacturer now advises the user that the two-

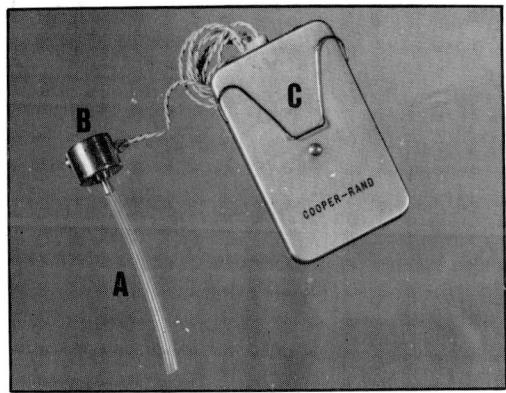

Figure 7-8. Cooper-Rand electronic larynx. A. Mouth tube. B. Hand-held tone generator. C. Pulse generator and battery case.

pronged cords can be plugged into the hand-held transducer in only one direction. Plugging in the cord in reverse results in an impedance mismatch and a noticeable reduction in loudness. The Cooper-Rand is available from Luminaud, P.O. Box 257, 7670 Acacia Avenue, Mentor, Ohio 44060, at an approximate cost of $175.00. The instrument uses two batteries (Eveready 411) which cost about $1.35 each.

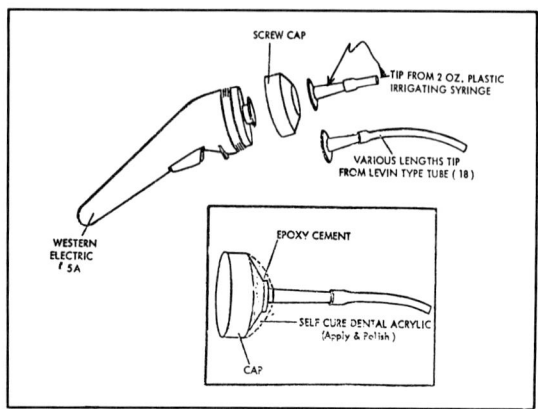

Figure 7-9. Mouth-type Western Electric No. 5 electronic larynx modification by Creech.

Modifications of the Western Electric No. 5 Electronic Larynx

Creech* recently described a simple and inexpensive modification of a standard Western Electric No. 5 neck-type electronic larynx into a mouth-type instrument (see Figure 7-9). The tapered tip of a 2-ounce plastic irrigating syringe is cemented with epoxy over the screw-on cap of a Western Electric No. 5, thereby enclosing the sound transducer. Dental acrylic is then applied around the circumference of the cap to further secure the syringe tip and to enhance the appearance of the instrument. This modified electronic larynx, either with or without a short piece of plastic tubing attached to the end of the syringe tip, is used in a manner similar to any other mouth-type artificial larynx. With the purchase of extra screw-on caps from the Bell Telephone Company (approximately $4.00 each), the modified instrument can easily be switched back to a neck-type instrument by simply replacing the modified cap with a standard cap. An unmodified Western Electric No. 5 artificial larynx can be purchased from the Bell Telephone Company at an approximate cost of $60.00.

* H. B. Creech 1976: personal communication.

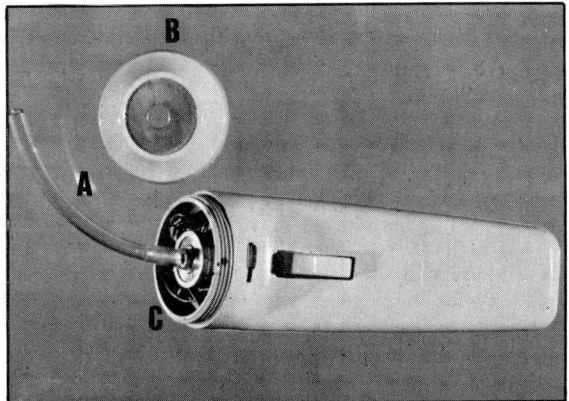

Figure 7-10. Mouth-type Western Electric No. 5 electronic larynx modification by Williams and Ostroy. A. Mouth tube. B. Screw-on cap with aluminum cover-plate. C. Body-type hearing aid receiver.

Williams and Ostroy* have developed a unique mouth-type electronic larynx using a Western Electric No. 5 as the basic unit. Their modification consists of replacing the standard transducer with a conventional hearing aid receiver (Figure 7-10). An aluminum cover-plate is used to stabilize the plastic mouth-tube which fits over the nub of the hearing aid receiver. This modified instrument produces a tone which is almost totally devoid of extraneous noise radiating from the head of the unit. Another important feature of this modification is that battery drain is decreased significantly (0.2 watts drain versus 1.5 watts). If the original transducer is saved, the instrument can be modified back into a neck-type electronic larynx when desired.

According to Williams:*

> The modification consists of removing the complete vibrating diaphragm unit and replacing it with a standard body-type hearing aid receiver. The receiver acts as a transducer, a speaker. The hearing aid receiver is glued securely in place within the space originally occupied by the vibrating diaphragm. The two wires from the Western Electric No. 5 circuit and the two short (unbraided) wires from the hearing aid receiver cord are soldered together, using the basic unit that supplies the energy to activate the hearing aid receiver. The electrical circuit of the Western Electric No. 5 is retained unless a small optional modification is desired. A 10K resistor can be connected in series with the variable tone control and 910K resistors in order to eliminate cut-off of

---

* W. G. Williams 1976: personal communication.

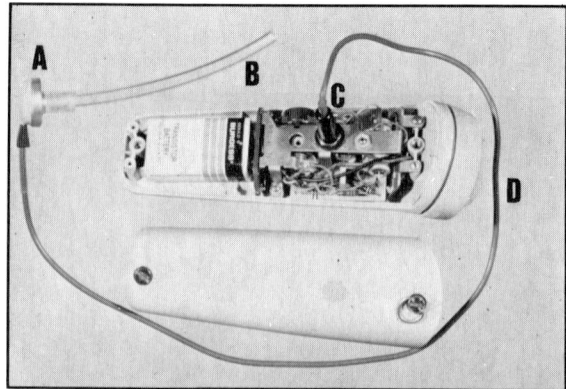

Figure 7-11. Mouth-type Western Electric No. 5 electronic larynx modification by Zwitman and Disinger. *A.* Body-type hearing aid receiver. *B.* Mouth tube. *C.* Shorting jack and plug. *D.* Cord.

the tone oscillator at its highest frequency. A three-inch piece of tygon tubing is fitted over the nub of the hearing aid receiver. An aluminum cover-plate is cut and fitted into the opening of the screw-on cap that previously accommodated the head of the vibrating diaphragm assembly. A hole is drilled in the center of the aluminum cover-plate large enough to allow the tygon tubing to slip freely through. The completed *cover* is then screwed down snugly to the body of the Western Electric No. 5. The final product is well-finished and attractive.

Zwitman and Disinger[14] reported a modification that consists of inserting a bypass plug into the circuitry of a Western Electric No. 5 electronic larynx, to convert it into a mouth-type instrument. The modified device consists basically of a standard neck-type transducer, a bypass plug, a cord leading to a hand-held body-type hearing aid receiver, and a plastic mouth-tube (see Figure 7-11). The instrument permits the user to select either mouth-type or neck-type use.

Knox* explained how to make the modification. The Zwitman modification is possible by a theoretically simple but technically exasperating addition of a shorting jack to the main frame of the device, which shunts the power from the output transducer to a hearing aid transducer when the alternate output plug is inserted in the jack.

As shown in Figure 7-11, the jack is located directly opposite the control knob, where according to Knox it does not interfere with the user's grip. It can be fastened on the main frame, and therefore wiring between the main frame and the removable back is not necessary. A hole is cut into the removable back to receive the plug from the mouth-type transducer. The

* A. Knox 1977: personal communication.

miniature shorting jack is typical of those used for personal speakers on transistor radios. The main frame is drilled and reamed out carefully to receive the threaded sleeve of the jack encased from both sides of the chassis by extruded fiber washers for electrical isolation. The red lead is then cut and wired both to the sleeve of the jack and to its power source. The normally closed terminal of the jack is wired to the green lead of the conventional Western Electric No. 5 transducer. The connection between them is opened when the plug is inserted, and output is routed to the hearing aid transducer. The conventional output transducer as measured on an impedance bridge has 20 ohms impedance at 1 KHz. A 15 ohm Telex RTR-04 hearing aid receiver is used because of the closeness of the impedance and the heavy-duty cord. A miniature plug is put on the cord replacing the $\frac{1}{4}$-inch standard plug.

The plastic mouth-tube can be any soft plastic tube with an adaptor to a $\frac{1}{4}$-inch interior dimension. In a demonstration instrument, a tube from a disposable plastic nasal cannula (Hudson No. 1102) was used by cutting off part of the slip-on adaptor for the oxygen tank. The thick, soft plastic wall worked very well. When the plug was inserted in the jack, the instrument became a mouth-type device; when it was removed, the instrument reverted to a neck-type artificial larynx.

AUREX NEOVOX M-550 INTRA-ORAL CONVERSION

Recently the Aurex Corporation made an adaptation kit available which permits easy conversion of the Aurex Neovox neck-type electronic larynx into a mouth-type device (Figure 7-12). The kit consists of a hard rubber cap and a plastic mouth-tube for collecting sound and conveying it into the mouth. This conversion results in a very satisfactory instrument

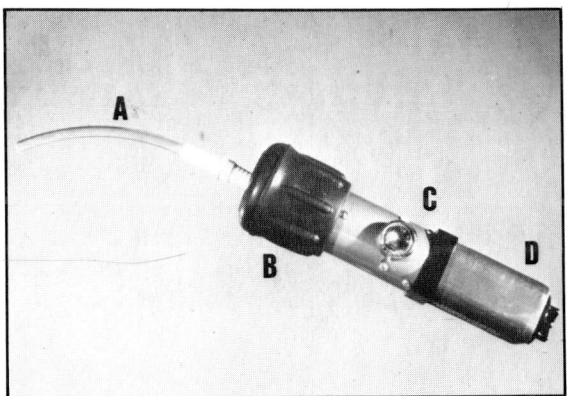

Figure 7-12. Aurex Neovox M-520T intra-oral conversion M-550. *A.* Mouth tube. *B.* M-550 cap. *C.* Vibrator mechanism. *D.* Rechargeable battery.

which is adequately devoid of extraneous noise. Intra-oral conversion kit M-550 can be purchased for approximately $15.00 from the Aurex Corporation, 844 West Adams Street, Chicago, Illinois 60607.

TICCHIONI PIPE

For many years a mouth-type electronic larynx concealed in a tobacco pipe, called "Pipa Di Ticchioni" after its developer, has been available in Europe (Figure 7-13). The present model has the battery attached to the base of the pipe bowl. A switch on the side of the bowl activates an internal tone generator and the sound produced is transmitted down the pipe stem to the user's mouth. The Ticchioni pipe is available from Ticchioni Ricerche Scientifiche Elettroiche, Via Pestalizzi 3E5 50018, Scandicci (Firenze) Italy, for approximately $300.00.

VERBALIZER VOICE SYNTHESIZER

The Verbalizer Voice Synthesizer is a mouth-type electronic larynx similar to the Cooper-Rand artificial larynx (Figure 7-14). The unit is a pocket-sized case which contains battery-powered circuitry connected by a cord to a hand-held transducer (body-type hearing aid receiver). Sound produced by the transducer enters the mouth via a small rubber tube. The Verbalizer is available from Cardwell Associates Inc., P.O. Box 1135, Torrance, California 90505, for approximately $225.00.

Electronic Neck-Type Artificial Larynges

WESTERN ELECTRIC 5A AND 5B ELECTRONIC LARYNGES

The most popular neck-type electronic larynx is probably the Western Electric 5A (low pitch for male) and 5B (high pitch for female). This instrument is a hand-held, battery-powered transducer that transmits sound into

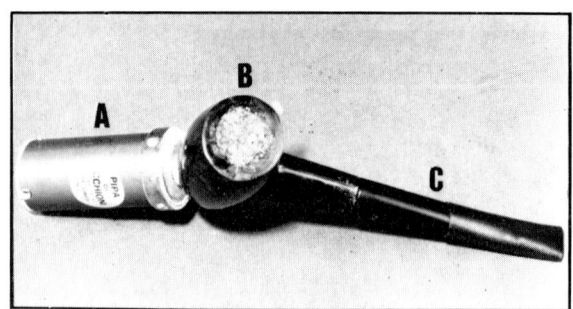

Figure 7-13. Ticchioni pipe artificial larynx. A. Battery. B. Pipe bowl containing tone generator. C. Pipe stem.

THE ARTIFICIAL LARYNX: PAST AND PRESENT

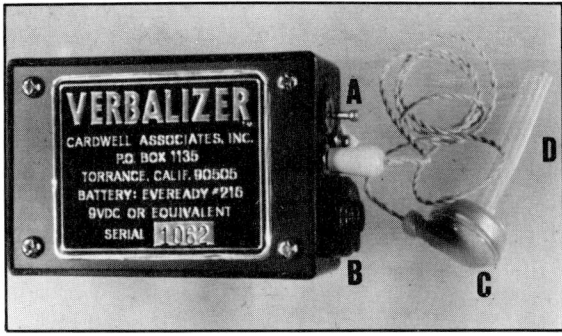

Figure 7-14. Verbalizer Voice Synthesizer. A. Tone activation switch. B. Volume control. C. Body-type hearing aid transducer. D. Mouth tube.

the resonance tract when correctly placed against the neck (Figure 7-15). Correct placement varies among users and must be determined by experimentation. It may be the midline junction between the neck and the floor of the mouth, the anterolateral aspect of the neck, or even the side of the face in instances when no suitable spot can be found on the neck and a mouth-type instrument is not available. For users who at first find it difficult to consistently find the appropriate spot on the neck, a piece of tape on the predetermined spot may help considerably.

The Western Electric No. 5 has an external variable pitch control incorporated in the on–off tone activation switch. The internal pre-set pitch range of the instrument can be adjusted to meet individual preference by

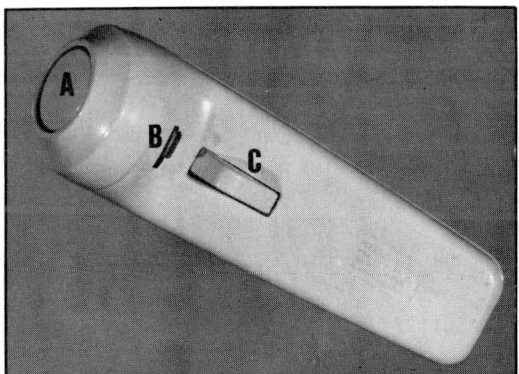

Figure 7-15. Western Electric No. 5 electronic larynx. A. Electromagnetic transducer. B. Power switch. C. Pitch control and on–off tone activation switch.

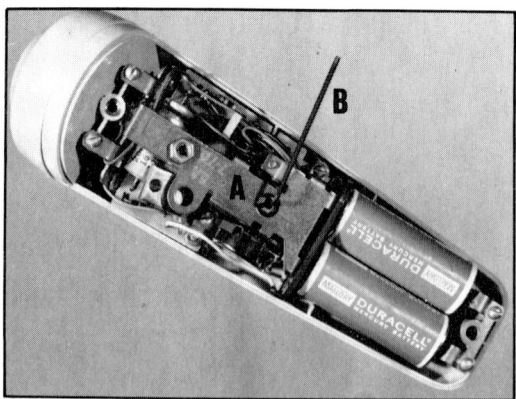

Figure 7-16. Preparing to adjust pitch range on the Western Electric No. 5 by loosening set screw A. with allen wrench B.

loosening a set screw with an allen wrench (Figure 7-16) and slowly adjusting a nearby screw while operating the instrument (Figure 7-17). Caution must be exercised when retightening the set screw to assure that the tone activation switch (variable pitch button), which is kept centered in its slot by the set screw, is centrally positioned before tightening. There is no provision for loudness variation. Extraneous noise radiating from the head of the instrument can be reduced by unscrewing the cap and packing a sound-absorbing material in the space around the transducer. Decreasing the degree to which the cap is screwed on (by about one and one-half turns) also seems to reduce extraneous vibratory noise in exceedingly loud instruments.

The Western Electric 5A and 5B can be purchased from the Bell

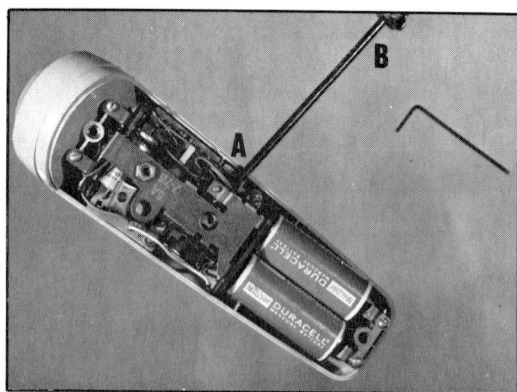

Figure 7-17. Adjusting Western Electric No. 5 pitch adjustment screw A. with a screw driver B.

THE ARTIFICIAL LARYNX: PAST AND PRESENT   75

Telephone Company at an approximate cost of $60.00. Inoperable instruments can be returned to the local telephone company at any time and will be replaced for a charge of approximately $5.00. The Western Electric No. 5 operates on two batteries (Eveready 164, Mallory TR164, Burgess H164, or RCA 164) that have a retail cost of approximately $3.75 each.

    A little known and relatively simple modification to the battery compartment of the Western Electric No. 5 electrolarynx can markedly alleviate battery cost and availability. The modification consists of slightly altering the battery compartment so that it will accept one standard 9-volt battery (Fig. 7-18). Figure 7-18 (A) shows the instrument unmodified. By unscrewing the metal clip and cutting off the two centered points of plastic in the floor of the case (B), the empty battery compartment (C) will accept a standard 9-volt battery (D). The battery should be carefully inserted (to avoid damage to contacts) so that the positive and negative terminals of the battery make good contact with corresponding electrical contacts in the battery case. It might be necessary to carefully pry these metal contacts slightly forward to insure firm contact with the terminals of the battery. If necessary, a small piece of foam rubber or tissue paper can be packed in the battery compartment to eliminate battery movement.

    With normal use a 9-volt battery will last eight to ten days. Although this is only one third as long as the two standard 5.6-volt batteries, three replacements of the 9-bolt battery per month only cost $2.75 ($.75 each). Even the better grade of alkaline 9-volt batteries only retail for $1.25 each for a total of $3.75 for three replacements each month. Monthly replacement of the two standard 5.6 volt batteries can cost from $5.50 to $10.00. Equally significant is the fact that 9-volt batteries are readily available at any drugstore or supermarket, and the standard 5.6-volt batteries are frequently difficult to procure.

    Popular brand-name 9-volt batteries and their respective model number are: Mallory MN 1604 (alkaline), Eveready 522 (alkaline). Mallory M1604, Burgess 2U6, Eveready 216, and Ray-O-Vac 1604. Assessment of battery-life characteristics has revealed that the alkaline 9-volt batteries (Mallory MN 1604, Eveready 522) last longer than the carbon zinc batteries. Cheap nonbrand-name 9-volt batteries should be avoided since they frequently have a short battery life. Recently introduced rechargeable nickel-cadmium 9-volt size batteries cannot be used in the Western Electric No. 5 electrolarynx without considerable compartment modification to accomodate their slightly larger size.

BARTS VIBRATOR ELECTRONIC LARYNX

    One of the newest neck-type electronic larynges available in the United States is the Barts Vibrator (Figure 7-19). This instrument basically consists of a small, battery-powered motor that drives a spring-loaded piston

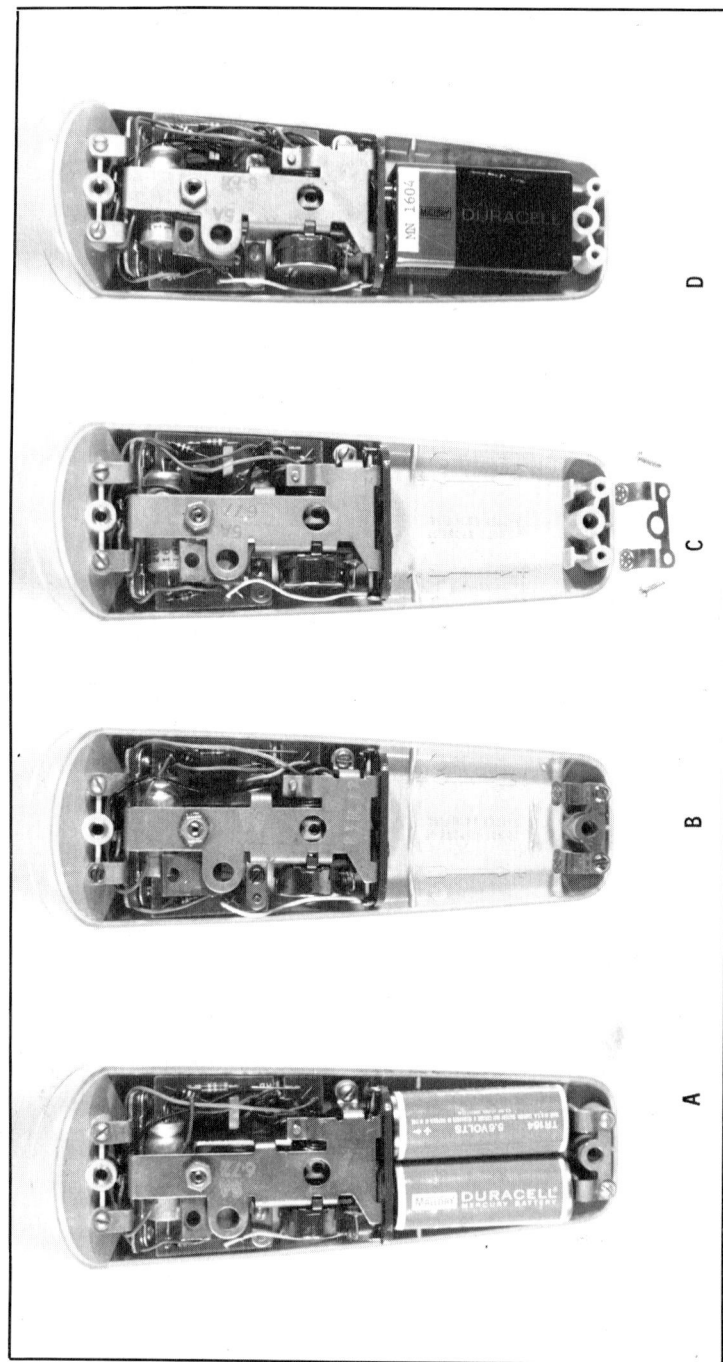

Figure 7-18. Conversion of the Western Electric No. 5 electronic larynx to a 9-volt power supply. A. Artificial larynx with two standard batteries. B. Remove metal clip and two centered points of plastic. C. Metal clip and two centered points of plastic removed. D. Artificial larynx with single 9-volt battery.

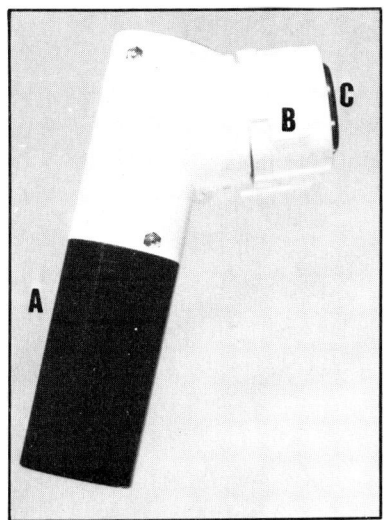

Figure 7-19. Barts Vibrator electronic larynx. *A.* Battery in handle. *B.* Locking ring. *C.* Vibrator mechanism.

against a diaphragm and thus produces sound. The mechanism is housed in a lightweight cylindrical case with an angled vibrator head. The loudness of the instrument is fixed, but pitch can be pre-set by adjusting a locking ring around the head of the vibrator. The Barts Vibrator is available from Park Surgical Company Inc., 5001 New Utrecht Avenue, Brooklyn, New York 11219, at an approximate cost of $195.00.

AUREX "NEOVOX" ELECTRONIC LARYNX

The Aurex "Neovox" M-520T is a battery-powered instrument that produces sound by means of a piston striking a diaphragm (Figure 7-20). The Aurex has an on–off tone activation switch with a ring around it that can be rotated to adjust loudness to a desired level. Although the manufacturer advises against altering the chrome collar that is located around the vibrating head of the instrument, minor alterations (less than one turn) do result in noticeable pitch variation. Under no circumstances should the cap be removed. The Aurex "Neovox" can be purchased from the Aurex Corporation, 844 West Adams Street, Chicago, Illinois 60607, for approximately $200.00. It uses an alkaline manganese battery 4E91 that can be purchased from the Aurex Corporation for approximately $2.50. A battery charger can also be purchased for approximately $45.00, and rechargable batteries for $20.00 each.

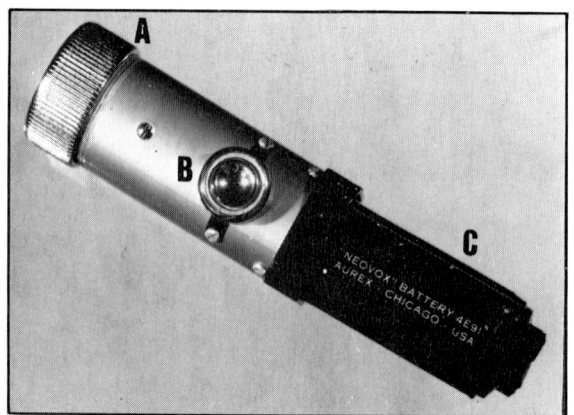

Figure 7-20. Aurex "Neovox" M-520T electronic larynx. A. Chrome collar around vibrator mechanism. B. On–off tone activation switch. C. Battery.

SERVOX ELECTRONIC LARYNX

The Siemens Servox is a high-quality German instrument (Figure 7-21). Sound is produced when a piston strikes a fixed diaphragm at a high velocity. The best quality of sound can be achieved by rotating the screw cap in which the diaphragm is mounted until the piston barely strikes this diaphragm at its farthest point of contact. Pitch and loudness may be

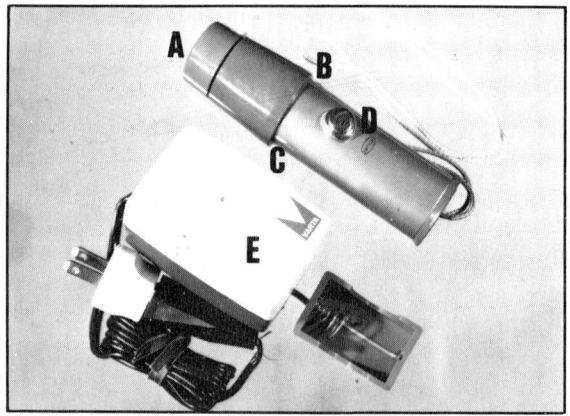

Figure 7-21. Siemen Servox electronic larynx. A. Vibrator mechanism. B. Pitch control switch. C. Volume control switch. D. On–off tone activation switch. E. Battery charger.

adjusted by rotating individual-function switches. Additionally, minimal pitch variation (5 to 20 Hz) can be achieved while talking by applying increased pressure to the tone activation switch. The Servox can be purchased from the Siemens Corporation, 186 Wood Avenue, Iselin, New Jersey 08830, at an approximate cost of $395.00. A rechargeable battery and battery charger are supplied with the instrument.

EMERGING SURGICAL-PROSTHETIC APPROACHES

In recent years there has been considerable interest in surgical reconstruction, both with and without incorporation of a prosthesis, as an approach to post-laryngectomy voice restoration. Prominent investigators who have contributed to this important area include Conley[15,16] Asai,[17] Montgomery and Toohill,[18,19] Taub and associates,[20-22] Shedd,[23] Komorn and associates,[24,25] Sisson,[26] McConnel et al.,[27] Edwards,[28-30] Serafini,[31] Arslan,[32,33] and Vega.[34] In this section the approaches of Taub, Shedd, and Sisson are briefly described. Their approaches toward surgical-prosthetic alaryngeal speech restoration currently appear to be undergoing either final-stage refinement or actual clinical application in the United States.

In 1972 Taub[20] described a combination surgical and prosthetic approach to vocal restoration for laryngectomees. Taub's surgical technique consists principally of a modified cervical esophagostomy. A longitudinal incision that parallels the lower anterior border of the sternocleidomastoid muscle is carried deeply between the sternal and clavicular heads of the anterior sheath into the retroesophageal space. The esophagus is exposed and an opening about the size of the tip of the fifth finger is created. The site of this opening is predetermined to assure that it will be below an esophageal segment suitable for phonatory vibration, but not so low that air will be directed into the stomach. The sternal head of the sternocleidomastoid muscle is severed and rotated around the carotid vessels as a bulky protective sheath. A superior-based skin flap of 9 cm in length and 7 cm in width is raised from the lateral aspect of the original incision, tubulated with the skin surface inwards and directed retrograde for a distance of approximately 5 cm, and sutured to the circumference of the opening in the esophagus. The donor-flap defect in the inferior aspect of the neck is closed by approximation of local tissue. A 26 Bardex tube is inserted in the fistula as a stent to assure fistula tract patency.

After satisfactory wound healing, usually 3 to 4 weeks, the external air-bypass prosthesis is interposed between the tracheostoma and the newly created fistula (Figure 7-22). The prosthesis consists chiefly of an adjustable

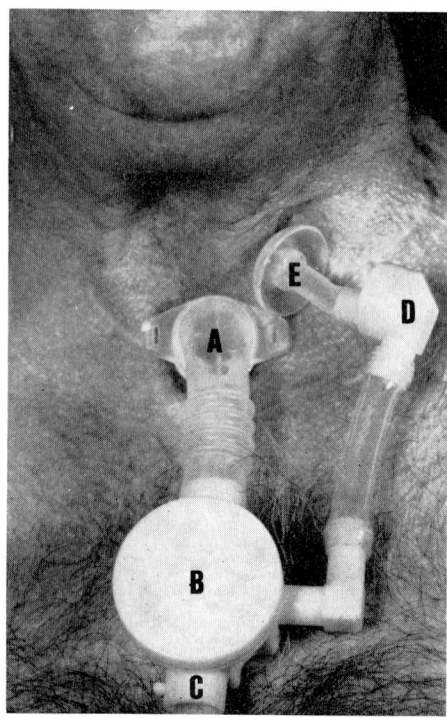

Figure 7-22. LaBarge VoiceBak prosthesis. A. Tracheal interconnector. B. Air-bypass flapper valve mechanism. C. Adjustable breathing port. D. One-way fistula valve. E. Flanged silastic fistula tube with tension collar. (Courtesy of LaBarge, Inc., St. Louis, Missouri)

differential valve capable of directing pulmonary air either out of the base of the prosthesis or through a side aperture which leads to the fistula in the esophagus. Differential valving is regulated by pulmonary breath pressure. Increased pulmonary breath pressure results in air being shunted into the esophagus and across approximated esophageal mucosa, thus creating vibratory excitation of the esophagus.

Blom[35] investigated acoustic and perceptual features of the speech of superior, highly trained esophageal speakers, and essentially untrained air-bypass speakers who previously had been unable to achieve functional esophageal speech through conventional instruction. The results of this investigation are summarized:

1. There were no significant group differences in average intelligibility between the esophageal and air-bypass speakers. The average intelligi-

bility for the six esophageal speakers and the six air-bypass speakers was 90 percent, as judged by both unsophisticated and sophisticated judges. The laryngectomized listeners reported somewhat lower speaker intelligibility scores; 79 percent for the air-bypass speakers and 83 percent for the esophageal speakers.
2. There were no significant differences in the ratings of average speaker acceptability between the two types of speakers as rated by any of the listener groups.
3. With respect to acoustic features, air-bypass speakers had a mean fundamental frequency of 69 Hz, with a range from 46 to 90 Hz. Average fundamental frequency for the esophageal speakers varied from 46 to 97 Hz, with a mean of 65 Hz.
4. Air-bypass speakers as a group spent 79 percent of their total speaking time producing periodic phonation, as compared to 63 percent for the esophageal speakers. The average time spent in aperiodic phonation was closely equivalent between the groups: 14 percent for the air-bypass group and 15 percent for the esophageal group. Silence consumed an average 7 percent of the air-bypass group's total speaking time. Esophageal speakers spent an average of 22 percent of their total speaking time in periods of silence.
5. With respect to duration characteristics for a 12-word sentence, air-bypass speakers as a group averaged 4.2 seconds. Individual speaker-time ranged from 3.4 to 4.8 seconds. Esophageal speakers as a group averaged 4.7 seconds, with individual speaker-times ranging from 3.7 to 6.6 seconds.
6. Average speaking rates for a 90-word passage were 141 words per minute for the air-bypass group and 157 words for the esophageal group.

Shedd[23] and his colleagues have been developing an experimental reed–fistula method of alaryngeal voice for patients who have undergone laryngo-pharyngectomy. The reed–fistula approach to speech restoration consists of interposing an external air-bypass and a pseudo-larynx mechanism between the tracheostoma and a surgically created pharyngeal fistula (Figure 7-23). The vibratory source for voice is essentially a modified Tokyo artificial larynx. This external sound source is excited and regulated by pulmonary air directed from the tracheostoma. Sound produced by the vibratory mechanism is transmitted to the vocal tract by a fistula tube.

Speech characteristics of the reed–fistula approach are reported by Weinberg et al.[36] and summarized here:

1. Average speech intelligibility for vowel materials ranges from 67 to 92 percent correct with an overall average intelligibility of 83 percent.

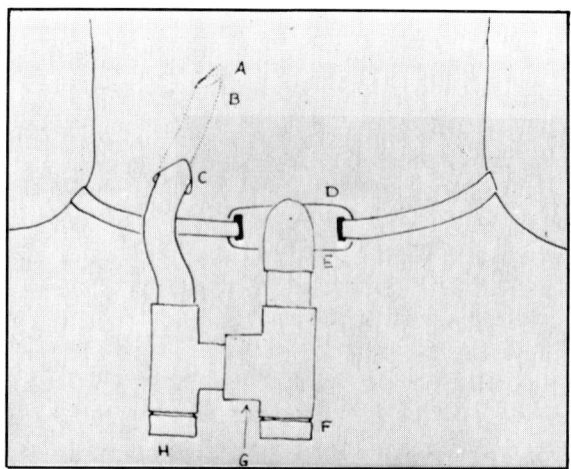

Figure 7-23. Diagram of reed–fistula speech appliance. A. Inner valve. B. Fistula tube in pharynx. C. Fistula opening. D. Tracheostomy tube. E. Tracheal connector. F. Inspiratory valve. G. Reed housing. H. Saliva trap. (Reprinted with permission. American Journal of Surgery 124:513, 1972.)

Average intelligibility for consonant elements ranges from 83 to 93 percent correct with an average overall intelligibility of 88 percent.
2. Fundamental frequency characteristics range from 107 Hz to 204 Hz. The standard deviations of fundamental frequency are 1 to 2 semitones and reflect the perceived monotonicity of pitch variability in reed–fistula speech.
2. Regarding phonation time characteristics: Percentage of time spent producing periodicity ranges from 33 percent to 60 percent. Aperiodicity consumes 4 percent to 20 percent of total speaking time, and silence accounts for 30 to 59 percent.

The developers of the reed–fistula method stress that their approach is clearly experimental at this time, and that it is not ready for routine application. Numerous speech, physiological, and biomedical liabilities remain to be resolved.

The Northwestern Voice Prosthesis has come into being through the concern of Sisson and his colleagues[26,27] for vocal restoration in patients who have undergone extensive resection and full-course radiation. These patients frequently are rendered poor candidates for either conventional methods of voice restoration or some of the other recently developed surgical-prosthetic approaches.

Sisson's vocal restoration approach usually takes advantage of a hypopharyngeal fistula that is created as part of the planned surgical approach to the patient's resection. This control fistula is constructed during resection in order to alleviate the potential formation of unplanned postoperative fistulas which frequently occur after extensive resection secondary to heavy preoperative radiation. Location of the control fistula varies from patient to patient. Of course, it is hoped that the fistula will enter below approximated tissue that is capable of being excited into audible vibration by shunted pulmonary air. According to Logemann[36] fluoroscopic studies have demonstrated that the vibratory source in talkers using the Northwestern Voice Prosthesis may be internal aspects of the fistula, a portion of the wall of the hypopharynx, the base of the tongue, or a combination of these structures. Fistulas that enter above tissue capable of being excited into vibration result in a whisper rather than true voice.

The Northwestern Voice Prosthesis consists basically of a tracheal connector, an adjustable pressure-sensitive respiratory valve, a conduit that leads to a one-way saliva valve which is designed to prevent reflux from entering the prosthesis, and a fistula fitting (Figure 7-24). The differential respiratory valve allows the patient to cough at very high expiratory pressure and to breathe normally at low pressures. The valve closes when expiratory breath pressure is slightly increased for speaking, and air is shunted through the prosthesis into the fistula and the vocal tract.

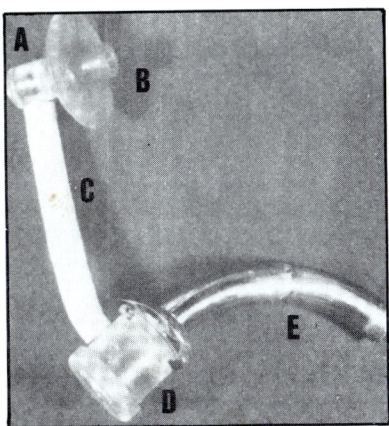

Figure 7-24. Northwestern Voice Prosthesis. A. One-way saliva valve. B. Fistula fitting. C. Conduit. D. Pressure-sensitive respiratory valve. E. Tracheal connector. (Reprinted with permission. Archives of Otolaryngology 101:179, 1975. Copyright 1975, American Medical Association.)

Results provided by Logemann on the speech of a small group of Northwestern Voice Prosthesis users are summarized here:

1. In a series of 13 speakers, eight had consistent voices and five had voices that were inconsistent. An inconsistent voice was defined as only being intermittently available to the speaker. In these speakers the source of vibration was usually the fistula, and its consistency was sometimes observed to vary with changes in head posture.
2. The voices of seven speakers revealed modal fundamental voice frequency that ranged from 87 Hz to 132 Hz with an average of 106 Hz. Individual speaker pitch variability ranged from a maximum of nine semitones to a minimum of four semitones.
3. Modal intensity for the seven speakers was in the range of 68 to 72 dB.
4. Ability to sustain voicing on a vowel varied among speakers. Three speakers sustained a vowel sound for 4 to 4.5 seconds and four speakers produced continuous voicing from 10 to 12 seconds.

Conclusion

This chapter has provided a review of artificial larynges, both past and present. To fully profit from the discussion of currently available artificial larynges, you are encouraged to obtain first-hand experience with each of the instruments. Become proficient at using them. Examine each artificial larynx available to you and learn how to make the adjustments and modifications described in this chapter. Listen to the accompanying cassette tape to increase your awareness of the sound produced by each type of instrument. With these exercises you will be better prepared to provide the laryngectomized with a second voice.

REFERENCES

1. Kallen LA: Vicarious vocal mechanisms: The anatomy, physiology and development of speech in laryngectomized persons. Arch Otolaryngol 20:460–503, 1934
2. Lebrun Y: The Artificial Larynx. Amsterdam, Swets and Zeitlinger BV, 1973
3. Arnold GE: Alleviation of alaryngeal phonation with the modern artificial larynx. I. Evaluation of artificial speech aids and their value for rehabilitation. Logos 3:55–67, 1960
4. Hanson WL: A new artificial larynx with a historical review. Ill Med J 78:483–486, 1940
5. McKesson EI: US Patent No 1,922,335 issued August 15, 1933
6. Riesz RR: US Patent No 1,910,966 issued May 23, 1933
7. Riesz RR: US Patent No 1,836,816 issued December 15, 1931

8. Cooper HK: US Patent No 2,862,209 issued December 2, 1958
9. Cooper HK, Millard RT: A dental approach to speech restoration in the laryngectomee. Dental Digest 65:106–112, 1959
10. Tait V, Tait RV: Speech rehabilitation with the oral vibrator. Speech Path Ther 2:64–69, 1959
11. Luchsinger R: Voice without a larynx: Alaryngeal dysphonia, in Luchsinger R, Arnold GE (eds): Voice–Speech–Language. Belmont, California, Wadsworth Publishing Co, 1949, p 288
12. Weinberg B, Riekena A: Speech produced with the Tokyo artificial larynx. J Speech Hearing Dis 38:383–389, 1973
13. Nelson IW, Parkin JL, Pottor JF: The modified Tokyo larynx. Arch Otolaryngol 101:107–108, 1975
14. Zwitman DH, Disinger JL: Experimental modification of the Western Electric #5 electrolarynx to a mouth-type instrument. J Speech Hearing Dis 40:35–39, 1975
15. Conley JJ, DeAmesti F, Pierce JK: A new surgical technique for the vocal rehabilitation of the laryngectomized patient. Ann Otol Rhinol Laryngol 67:655–664, 1958
16. Conley JJ: Vocal rehabilitation by autogenous vein graft. Ann Otol Rhinol Laryngol 68:990–995, 1959
17. Asai R: Laryngoplasty after total laryngectomy. Arch Otolaryngol 95:114–119, 1972
18. Montgomery WW, Toohill RJ: Voice rehabilitation after laryngectomy. Arch Otolaryngol 88:499–506, 1968
19. Montgomery WW: Postlaryngectomy vocal rehabilitation. Arch Otolaryngol 95:76–83, 1972
20. Taub S, Spiro RH: Vocal rehabilitation of laryngectomees: Preliminary report of a new technic. Am J Surg 124:87–90, 1972
21. Taub S, Bergner LH: Air bypass voice prosthesis for vocal rehabilitation of laryngectomees. Am J Surg 125:748–756, 1973
22. Taub S: Air bypass voice prosthesis for vocal rehabilitation of laryngectomees. Ann Otol Rhinol Laryngol 84:45–48, 1975
23. Shedd D, Bakamjian V, Sako K, et al: Reed-fistula method of speech rehabilitation after laryngectomy. Am J Surg 124:510–514, 1972
24. Komorn RM, Weycer JS, Sessions RB, et al: Vocal rehabilitation with a tracheo-esophageal shunt. Arch Otolaryngol 97:303–305, 1973
25. Komorn RM: Vocal rehabilitation in the laryngectomized patient with a tracheo-esophageal shunt. Ann Otol Rhinol Laryngol 83:445–451, 1974
26. Sisson GA, McConnel FMS, Logemann JA, et al: Voice rehabilitation after laryngectomy. Arch Otolaryngol 101:178–181, 1975
27. McConnel FMS, Sisson GA, Logemann JA: Three years' experience with a hypopharyngeal pseudoglottis after total laryngectomy. Trans Am Acad Ophthalmol Otolaryngol 84:63–67, 1977
28. Edwards N: Post-laryngectomy vocal rehabilitation. J Laryngol Otol 88:905–918, 1974
29. Edwards N: Post-laryngectomy rehabilitation by the external fistula method: Further experiences. Laryngoscope 85:690–699, 1975

30. Edwards N: New voices for old: Restoration of effective speech after laryngectomy by the pulmonary air shunt-vocal fistula principle. Bristol Medico Chirurgical J 90:11–17, 1976
31. Serafini I: A case of total laryngectomy with maintained natural breathing operated with a personal technique. Panminerva Med 13:377–386, 1971
32. Arslan M: Reconstructive laryngectomy: Report of the first 35 cases. Ann Otol Rhinol Laryngol 81:479–486, 1972
33. Arslan M: Techniques of laryngeal reconstruction. Laryngoscope 85:862–865, 1975
34. Vega MF: Larynx reconstruction surgery: A study of three-year findings: A modified surgical technique. Laryngoscope 85:866–881, 1975
35. Blom ED: A comparative investigation of acoustical and perceptual features of esophageal speech and speech with the Taub voice prosthesis, dissertation, College Park, Maryland, University of Maryland, 1972
36. Weinberg B, Logemann JA, Singer M, et al: Surgical prosthetic approaches to speech rehabilitation after laryngectomy: An overview. Third Annual Symposium on Vocal Rehabilitation of the Laryngectomized, Indianapolis, 1977

Howard B. Rothman, Ph.D.

8.
Analyzing Artificial Electronic Larynx Speech

Considerable amounts of effort and study have been expended in recent years to develop alternate modes of speech production for laryngectomized individuals. Specifically, investigators have explored alternate surgical techniques in combination with various forms of prosthetic appliances and devices for generating speech sounds. These include esophageal speech, air-bypass, pneumatic and electronic larynges, tracheo-esophageal shunts, and pharyngo-tracheal fistulas. The mode of speech production chosen by a laryngectomized individual is often dependent on several factors, such as health status, personal preference, the ability to learn esophageal speech, the ability to undergo secondary surgery, or willingness to tolerate and care for a prosthesis. Whatever primary mode of speech production is ultimately chosen, there is general agreement that at one time or another every laryngectomee may need to use an artificial larynx.

NORMAL SPEECH PRODUCTION

Before describing speech produced with an artificial larynx, a brief explanation of normal speech production will be useful. Stated very simply, speech is the product of sound sources (for example, the vibratory action of the vocal folds and constrictions or closures above the larynx) and the resonation of the vocal cavities (or tract) excited by these sources. The sound energy that activates the resonating properties of the vocal tract is provided by the vibratory action of the vocal folds and constrictions or closures above the larynx. In normal speech production, the vocal tract can be thought of as a series of interconnecting and complexly coupled resonating cavities. At one end the vocal tract is bound by the vibrating vocal folds; at the other end, the vocal tract terminates at the lips unless the nasal cavities are engaged in sound production.

Figure 8-1 is a schematic view of the human speech mechanism. In order to produce a speech sound, the air in the vocal tract must be excited or vibrated in some way. The three-dimensional aspects of the resonating system are altered through the contraction of muscles that regulate the movements of the articulators—the tongue, mandible (or jaw), lips and velum (or soft palate), as well as the pharynx, epiglottis, and larynx.

Speech sounds are generally classified into two broad categories: vowels and consonants. In normal speech production, vowels are called voiced sounds and are produced with a laryngeal sound source, that is, by the vibratory action of the vocal folds. This vibratory action sets the air coming from the lungs into motion, and this motion in turn passes through the vocal tract and radiates outward from the lips.

Consonant sounds may be voiced or voiceless. They are produced by constrictions or occlusions which occur above the level of the larynx in the vocal tract. The primary source of sound for a voiceless consonant is a constriction where air turbulence is created (for example, the /s/ sound), or a closure which causes a pressure build-up followed by a sudden release (for example, the /p/ sound). Certain sounds, such as the voiced fricative /v/ have two sound sources: the vibrating vocal folds and the turbulent air forced between the upper front teeth and the lower lip.

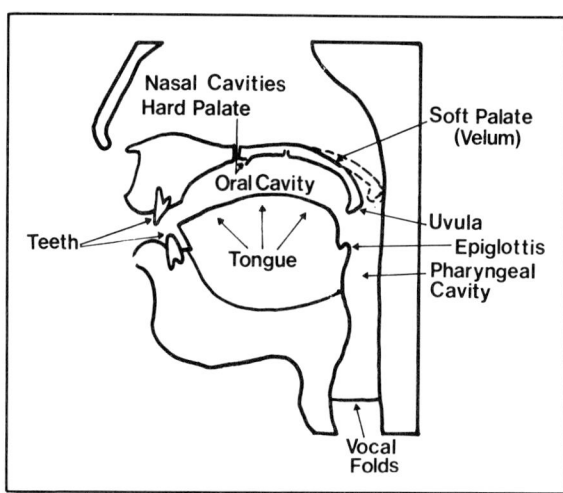

Figure 8-1. A schematic view of the human speech mechanism.

All speech sounds, whether they are vowels or voiced/voiceless consonants, share one common trait. They are produced by a vibratory motion—sometimes periodic or regular, and sometimes aperiodic or turbulent—that excites the resonating properties of the vocal tract. The resonating characteristics of the vocal tract are determined, at every instant in time, by the size and shape of the three-dimensional tube. The resulting acoustic (sound) output is characterized by a number of resonant peaks or formants which reflect the resonating characteristics of the vocal tract at any given moment.

ARTIFICIAL LARYNX SPEECH

The artificial larynx has been available in various forms for over 100 years. In fact, the first successful human laryngectomy was performed in 1873 by the great Viennese surgeon, Theodore Billroth, a friend of the composer Brahms. As Blom stated in Chapter 7, the first artificial larynx was a pneumatic prosthesis. The first usable electronic artificial larynx was devised in 1942 and has remained relatively unchanged during the past 35 years.

Analysis of Artificial Larynx Speech

In a presentation to the Pacific Coast Oto-Ophthalmological Society in 1974, Byron Bailey[1] expressed the view that new ideas and approaches are needed. I strongly endorse that statement. Since that meeting most of the new ideas and approaches have been surgical in nature. The success of these endeavors has been limited for various reasons. Further, many laryngectomees may be unable or unwilling to undergo an additional surgical procedure.

Bailey and Goode[2] in 1975 stated that the laryngectomee should first be encouraged to develop esophageal or electronic laryngeal speech. Yet it is generally conceded that approximately one-third of the laryngectomized population fails to acquire esophageal speech. Fully one-half of those laryngectomees aged sixty years and older cannot learn to utilize the esophageal method.[3] It is doubtful that this population would be considered prime candidates for techniques requiring further voice-restoration surgery. Therefore, when the total population of laryngectomees is considered, it is important that a simple and relatively inexpensive method of producing intelligible and acceptable speech be made available. At present the most widely used approach involves a neck-type artificial larynx. Perhaps at this time a point made earlier should be reemphasized: at one time or another, the use of an artificial larynx is necessary for virtually all laryngectomees.

The remainder of this chapter is concerned with analyzing speech produced with such devices.

The scientific literature concerning the neck-type artificial larynx is relatively sparse and primarily is concerned with comparing artificial larynx speech to esophageal and normal speech. Information that compares good and poor esophageal speakers can be used for establishing standardized criteria for esophageal speech. However, there is virtually no information that compares good or poor artificial larynx speakers. Thus we have relatively little data with which to establish standards and criteria for evaluation of artificial larynx speech, and for determining when to terminate treatment. In fact, before it is possible to compare the speech of good and poor electronic larynx users, the degree of speech proficiency categorizing the two groups must be determined.

DETERMINING SPEECH COMMUNICATION PROFICIENCY: PART I

In a study conducted by Goldstein and Rothman,[4] 15 artificial larynx speakers were tape-recorded while reading eight CID everyday sentences. These sentences were prepared at the Central Institute for the Deaf to represent everyday American speech. The specifications were determined by a working group of the Armed Forces National Research Council Committee on Hearing and Bio-Acoustics. Among the criteria they deemed important for these sentences were low abstraction level, high redundancy, a vocabulary appropriate for adults, utilization of words that occur with high frequency, and finally, usage of contractions and nonslang idioms. The grammatical structure of the CID sentences vary, as does sentence length. The types of sentence forms used are declarative, imperative, rising interrogative, and falling interrogative.[5]

Recording procedures utilized by Goldstein and Rothman[4] followed well-established standards to insure that the recording itself would not become a variable affecting listener judgments. Six experienced speech pathologists rated each speaker's speech communication proficiency on a 7-point, equal-appearing interval scale. A 1 represented "least proficient" and 7 represented "most proficient." The ratings were based on each speech pathologist's experience of what constitutes speech communication proficiency. The inter-judge reliability of averaged ratings was 0.76, which indicated that the six speech pathologists were utilizing similar criteria in their judgments. The ratings given to each speaker were averaged and the averaged scores then were used to assign each speaker into one of three groups. The group of five highest-scoring speakers (mean proficiency rating of 6.33) and the group of five lowest-scoring speakers (mean proficiency rating of 2.73) were used for comparison purposes. A nonparametric test was used to confirm the difference between the two groups at the .001 level.[4]

All of the laryngectomees used neck-type electronic larynges. Seven of them used a Western Electric No. 5 and the remaining three used an Aurex Neovox. The five laryngectomees comprising the poor speaker group were, on the average, five years older than the good speakers (68 versus 63 years) and they also averaged 1.6 years less formal education. The average length of time from surgery to date of recording was seven years. None of the speakers were involved at the time in speech treatment. As a point of interest, the poor speakers on the average had had 1.2 hours more speech treatment than the good speakers.

ANALYSIS OF FREQUENCY, SPEECH RATE, AND INTENSITY

After establishing the two groups of artificial electronic larynx speakers, the following speech parameters were chosen for measurement and analysis.

1. Frequency range of the vibratory pulses of the electronic artificial larynges.
2. Speech rate.
3. Intensity.

These parameters were initially chosen in order to determine whether rate of speech, intensity variations and pitch manipulations differentiated the two groups, and also if they were related to the proficiency ratings. The results of the ratings and measurements can be seen in Table 8-1.

Frequency range. Measurements of frequency range were obtained by using a Honeywell 1508A Visicorder, which is an oscillograph with a paper read-out indicating frequency and amplitude. The 12-word sentence, "How do you feel about changing the time when be begin to work?" was used to determine the range of frequencies. The speakers in the poor group were able to vary pitch from 6.61 to 15.32 Hz, with a mean range of 11.10 Hz. The good speakers used frequency ranges of 13.06 to 20.26 Hz, with a mean range of 16.10 Hz.

The nonparametric Mann-Whitney U was used to test whether the frequency ranges utilized by the two groups were, in fact, significantly different. A U of 3 was obtained, indicating that the two groups were significantly different with a probability of .028. It is interesting to note that three of the ten speakers used an Aurex "Neovox" device, which does not contain a pitch variation control. These are speakers 4, 7, and 8 in Table 8-1.

Table 8-1.
Verbal Communication Proficiency Ratings and Measurements for Two Groups of Artificial Larnyx Speakers, and Results of a Mann-Whitney U Test Indicating the Significance of Differences Between the Two Groups.

	Proficiency Ratings	Rate of Speaking*	Intensity Range*	Frequency Range
Poor Speakers				
1	3.66	6.29	9.0	6.61
2	3.66	4.26	18.1	7.46
3	2.50	4.53	27.3	12.72
4	2.50	6.95	8.3	15.32
5	1.33	10.37	4.5	13.41
Means	2.73	6.48	13.4	11.10
S.D.	0.87	2.23	8.2	3.42
Good Speakers				
6	6.33	4.28	22.7	20.26
7	6.33	3.25	113.6	14.13
8	6.33	3.95	45.7	16.69
9	5.83	4.14	12.0	16.38
10	6.50	3.70	45.5	13.06
Means	6.33	3.86	47.9	16.10
S.D.	.28	.36	31.6	2.48
Mann-Whitney U	0	1	3	3
P =	.001	.008	.028	.028

* Rate of speaking was measured in seconds; intensity was measured in Hertz (Hz).

As can be seen in the table, they were able to achieve frequency ranges comparable to those using the Western Electric No. 5, which does have a pitch variation control.

Speech rate. As shown in Table 8-1, the time necessary for the poor speakers to utter the 12-word sentence ranged from 4.26 to 10.37 seconds, with a mean rate of 6.48 seconds for the group. A speaking rate ranging from 3.25 to 4.28 seconds with a mean of 3.86 seconds was obtained by the good speakers. A Mann-Whitney U of 1 with a probability greater than .008 indicates that the good speakers were significantly different from the poor speakers. These data were compared with data concerning the speaking rate of esophageal speakers obtained by Curry and Snidecor,[6] Shipp,[7] and Bennett and Weinberg.[8] The esophageal speakers utilized in those investigations spoke with ranges of 5.4 to 6.0 seconds, or at a slower rate than the good artificial larynx speakers from this investigation.

Intensity. Table 8-1 also shows the ranges of intensity, measured in millivolts, used by the two groups. These intensity ranges were obtained with a Bruel and Kjaer Level Recorder. Three different sentences were used to obtain each speaker's intensity range. The intensity variation of the poor speakers ranged from 4.5 to 27.3 millivolts, with a mean of 13.4 millivolts. For the good speakers, it was from 12 to 113.6 millivolts, with a mean of 47.9 millivolts. The Mann-Whitney test indicates that the two groups were significantly different with a probability of .028.

Spearman Rank Correlation Coefficients were obtained to determine the relationship between each of the speech variables measured (that is, speaking rate, intensity range, and frequency range) to the proficiency ratings. As shown in Table 8-2, proficiency ratings and rate and intensity ranges are all significantly correlated at the .01 level. According to Table 8-2, the speech variable of rate is most highly correlated with the proficiency rating. As seen in Table 8-1, it was the speech rate variable that most significantly differentiated the two groups. Therefore speech rate appears to be the most powerful feature for indicating proficiency on the artificial larynx, at least for the speakers in this study. We expected that frequency range would be a distinguishing feature and it was not; evidently, the users of the Western Electric device did not utilize its variable pitch control effectively.

An obvious question at this point is: "How are pitch and intensity variations accomplished?" This question is especially germane in regard to

Table 8-2.
Results of a Spearman Rank Correlation Coefficients Test.

	Spearman Rank Correlation Coefficients			
	Proficiency Ratings	*Rate of Speaking*	*Intensity Range*	*Frequency Range*
Proficiency Ratings	1.00	.94*	.77*	.47
Rate of Speaking	—	1.00	.86*	.21
Intensity Range	—	—	1.00	.18
Frequency Range	—	—	—	1.00

* P < .01

the Aurex "Neovox," which has no variable pitch control. The physical correlate of pitch is frequency. It is determined by the number of repetitive vibrations occurring per second. All the neck-type electronic larynges have a vibrating disc driven by some mechanical means, such as a piston. When the vibrating disc is pressed against the tissues of the neck and the pressure is slightly increased, a change occurs in the relationship between the disc and the piston. This change reduces the excursion of the piston and results in an intensity change. In turn, there may occur a differential loading effect on the electronics producing the pulse rate with which the piston is driven. Any alteration of the pulse rate also will affect the frequency or perceived pitch. Isshiki and Tanabe[9] discussed this damping effect on the high-frequency end of the spectrum.

Two additional variables that separate the two groups should be mentioned. Extraneous noises and pauses occur during the reading of the sentences. Extraneous noise occurs when a device is not completely coupled to the neck tissues. The poor speakers averaged two occurrences of extraneous noise while reading the eight sentences; the good speakers had none. The poor speakers averaged 3.2 inappropriate pauses (the device was, in effect, shut down) per sentence and the good speakers averaged only .48 pauses per sentence.

To summarize, speech rate and intensity range were highly correlated to ratings of speech or communication proficiency. Frequency variation, at least for these two groups, was not. Other indications of a good artificial larynx user, as opposed to a poor one, were the number of extraneous noises and inappropriate pauses involved in speaking.

DETERMINING SPEECH COMMUNICATION PROFICIENCY: PART II

In order to establish a more complete profile of communication proficiency, a further attempt was initiated to study other necessary parameters of speech. In 1976 Rothman and Goldstein[10] undertook a series of investigations to specify some of the aspects of duration and amplitude in the articulation of speech. They used the same population of good and poor speakers as previously described. The first part of this investigation has been completed and is discussed here.

Articulation

Articulation concerns the movement of tongue, lips, teeth, jaw, and soft palate. The movement of these organs and structures changes the configuration of the vocal tract and results in the formation of speech sounds. Articulation measures were made from spectrograms produced on a Voice Identification Series 700 Spectrograph. The sound spectrograph provides a graphic display of a signal, with time portrayed on the horizontal axis and frequency on the vertical axis. Vowel formants are defined as areas of acoustic energy maxima corresponding to the resonant frequencies of the vocal tract at any given moment in time. Formant transitions represent articulatory movement from the place of consonant production to the position of the adjacent vowel and vice versa. Vowel formants and formant transitions are seen on the spectrograph as horizontal or moving bars at different frequencies. Intensity differences appear as darker (greater intensity) or lighter bars. Figure 8-2 is an example of this kind of spectrogram, a wide-band spectrogram of the sentence "I don't want to go to the movies tonight," spoken by an adult male with a normal larynx.

Wide-band, bar-type spectrograms, and amplitude displays were made of the following three sentences:

1. I don't want *to go to* the movies tonight.
2. Do you think that she should stay *out so* late?
3. This suit needs *to go to* the cleaners.

These three sentences (from the original corpus of eight) were chosen because they contained a relatively large number of voiced and voiceless stop plosives and voiceless fricatives, classes of speech sounds whose production or within-class differentiation is often difficult for users of artificial larynges. The italicized words in the sentences above contain the phonological elements used for measurement purposes.

Measurements from the wide-band spectrograms included the following considerations.

For the plosives, the *stop-closure duration* was measured from the end of the preceding vocalic to the release of the stop, or in some cases to the beginning of the next vocalic. Vocalics are speech sounds whose energy source is vocal fold vibration; for example, vowels. In Figure 8-2 vocalics are the sounds with vertical striations. At times, measuring closure duration from vocalic to vocalic was indicated because some speakers never released the plosive. Rather, they appeared to implode the intervocalic stop, and tended to treat the voiceless stops as voiced. This voicing of intervocalic voiceless stops is not unusual in normal speakers.

In some cases that we measured we were forced to give a value of zero milliseconds to a closure because there was no observable stoppage or diminution of acoustic energy. That is, to simulate the silent interval or closure duration characteristic of articulatory closure for stop-consonants, the speaker would have to momentarily deactivate his device or dampen the intensity of the acoustic energy in some way. There was no evidence that

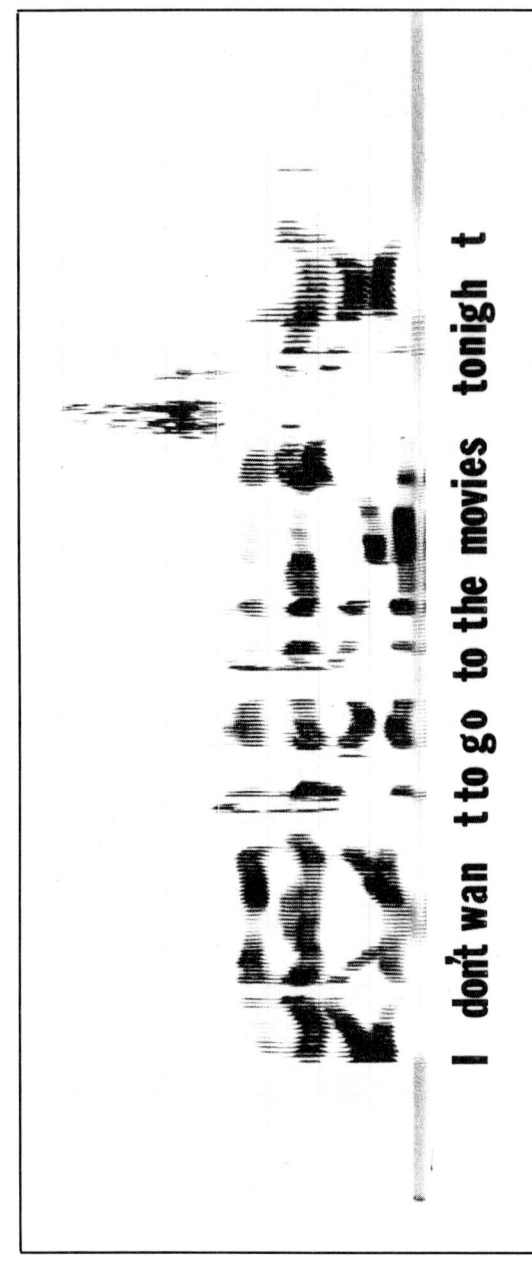

Figure 8-2. A wide-band spectrogram of the sentence, "I don't want to go to the movies tonight." The speaker is an adult male with a normal larynx.

this was done in the examples to which we assigned a value of zero milliseconds. In other cases a value of infinity milliseconds was assigned when a speaker obviously "shut down" completely during what should have been an articulatory closure. For example, several speakers, in effect, stopped talking and turned the artificial larynx off for as much as 250 milliseconds (¼ of a second) before continuing.

The *duration of fricatives* was measured for the length of observed frication. Sometimes the value of infinity milliseconds was also assigned for fricative duration because the speakers paused and omitted the fricative.

Relative intensity measurements were made from amplitude displays of each of the phonological segments cited previously. These measurements were undertaken to determine if artificial larynx users could attenuate the vibratory duty-cycle of their device in order to (a) differentiate between voiced/voiceless speech sounds; or (b) allow for approximations of closure durations for stop consonants.

RESULTS

The results of the measurements generally indicate that the two groups of artificial larynx speakers were significantly different on several articulatory parameters. These differences are summarized in Table 8-3. According to Table 8-3, duration and/or amplitude are significantly distinguishing features between the articulatory patterns of the two groups' production of the intervocalic voiceless stop / d /, voiced stop / t /, and the voiceless fricative / s /.

Table 8-3.
Results of Spearman Rank Correlations Test Relating Proficiency to Amplitude and Duration and Results of a Mann-Whitney U Test.

		Proficiency Ratings	Significant Differences
Go	D.	0.067	12
	A.	0.15	12
To	D.	0.54	7
	A.	0.68*	3*
Should	D.	0.59*	4*
	A.	0.36	11
Stay	D.	0.42	5.5
Outso	D.	0.82†	1†
	A.	0.71†	3*
Outso	D.	0.67*	4.5*

D. = Duration * = P < .05
A. = Amplitude † = P < .01

Therefore, the data strongly indicate that duration and amplitude of certain phonological elements distinguish between these good and poor artificial larynx users, and further, are related to rating the users' speaking proficiency.

The data also indicate less inter-speaker variation in the group of good speakers than in the group of poor speakers. For the stops and fricatives, the poor speakers were more likely to implode or stop phonation, or to omit frication during connected discourse. These omissions, implosions, or pauses result in the measurements ranging from zero to infinity especially for the poor speakers. Several examples illustrating these findings follow.

Figure 8-3 is a wide-band spectrogram of a good speaker saying " . . . to go to the movies tonight." First, notice the big gap before point A that indicates an inappropriate pause between the words "go" and "to." This gap was measured as infinity milliseconds. Following the gap is a sudden release of energy, called a spike (point A in the figure), indicating the sudden release of a broad-band burst of transient energy which is characteristic of a stop-consonant release. Following the spike and before the onset of voicing (in this case, the activation of the electronic larynx indicated by the vertical striations) is an appropriate voiceless release period with aspiration of approximately 50 milliseconds.

Obviously, the good artificial larynx speaker who produced this speech segment used buccal air—i.e., air trapped in the cheeks or mouth—to cause a pressure increase behind the tongue closure. On release of the trapped air, the speaker waited for the aspiration release period—shown between points A and B in Figure 8-3—before starting the electronic larynx for the next vocalic. At point C, middle to high frequency frication noticeably indicates the use of buccal air in the production of the final /z/ sound in "movies." Since /z/ is a voiced fricative, the speaker did not deactivate the electronic larynx. Point D is the spike release of the first /t/ in "tonight." The speaker again did not deactivate the electronic larynx. However, a slight pressure of the vibrating disc of the artificial larynx, lasting about 20 milliseconds, attenuated the vibratory cycle of the device and thereby enabled the slight aspiration of the release to be audible to listeners.

The following figures show wide-band spectrograms (Figure 8-4) and amplitude displays (Figure 8-5) of both a good and a poor speaker. The displays of the good speaker are at the top half of each figure. The utterance in both cases is "This suit needs to go to the cleaners." The figures are arranged in a way to facilitate visual comparisons between the good and poor speakers.

The most striking difference between the two spectrograms in Figure 8-4 can be seen by examining the presence of vertical striations, which indicate the vibratory duty cycle of the electronic larynx. The spectrogram of the poor speaker indicates that the electronic larynx was activated for the

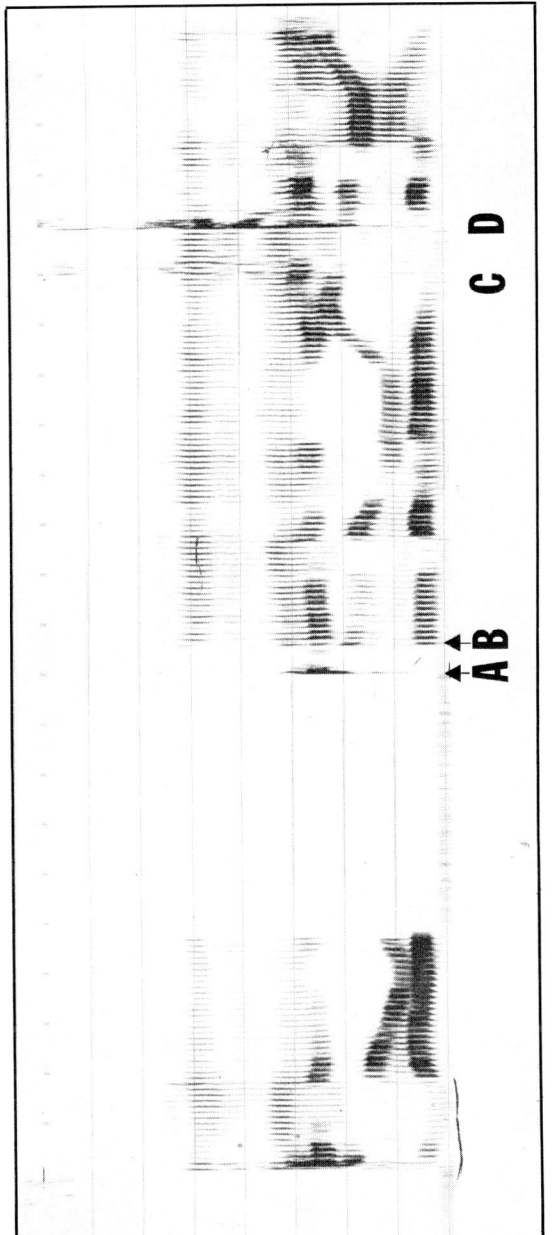

Figure 8-3. A wide-band spectrogram of a good artificial larynx speaker's production of "to go to the movies tonight." **A** indicates the release burst and aspiration of the /t/ following the word "go." There is an appropriate delay of approximately 50 ms before onset of the periodic artificial larynx buzz. **B** indicates the onset of the vocalic of the word "to." **C** indicates the /z/ in the word "movies," and **D** indicates the burst and aspiration of the first /t/ in "tonight." Notice that the aspiration at **D** is superimposed on the periodic artificial larynx buzz.

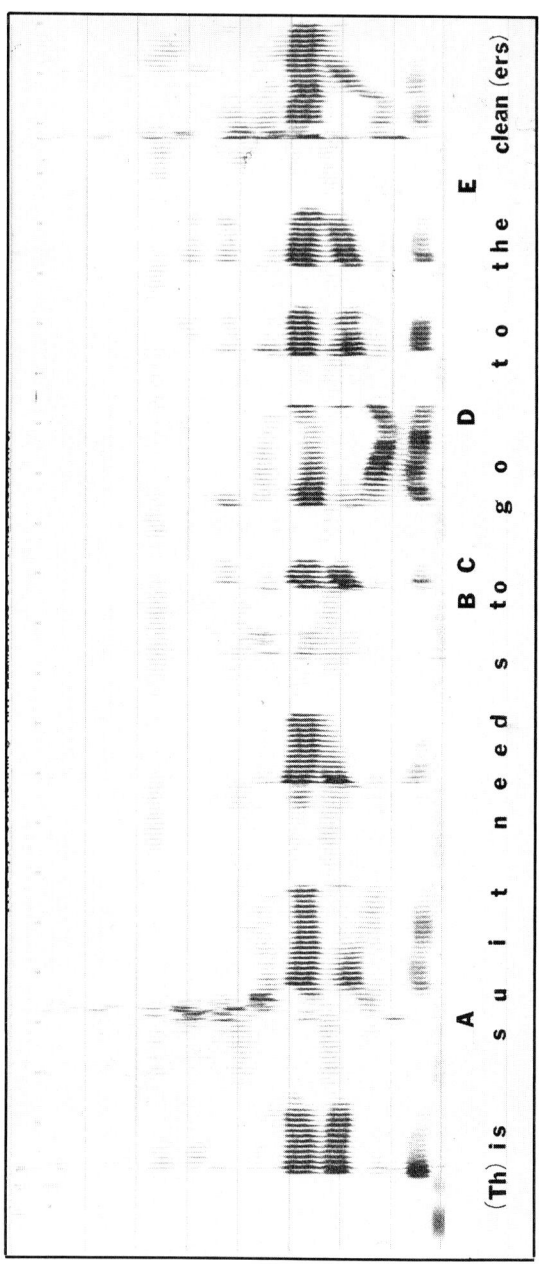

Figure 8-4 (top).

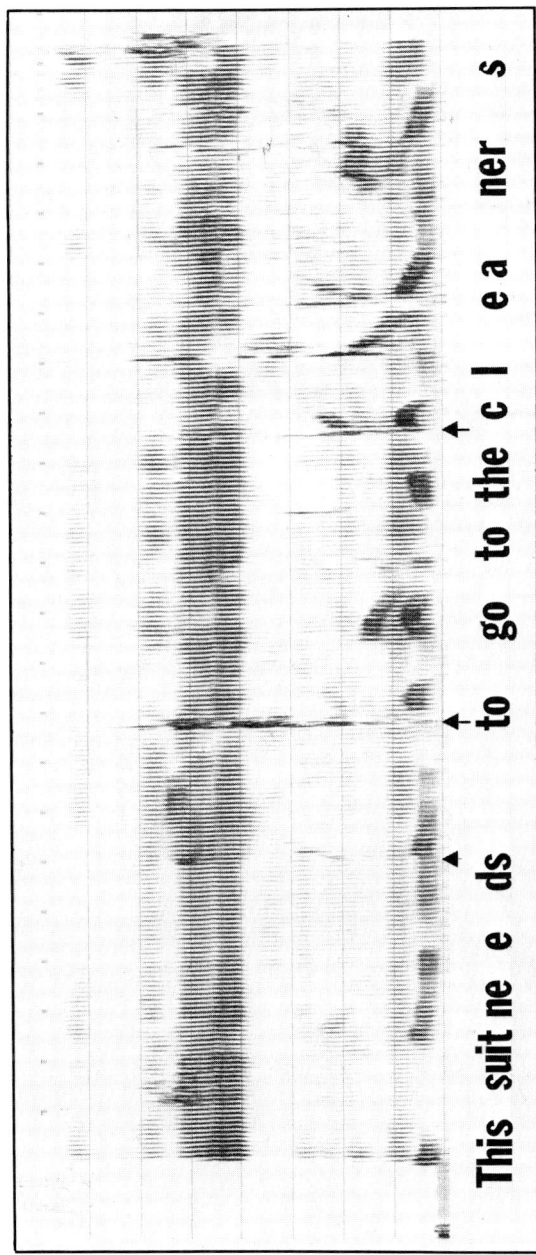

Figure 8-4 (*bottom*). Wide-band spectrograms of a good (*top*) and a poor (*bottom*) artificial larynx speaker's production of "This suit needs to go to the cleaners." The orthographic representation of the sentence is spaced to approximate the appearance of the associated acoustic events. Features highlighted by letters or arrows are explained in the text.

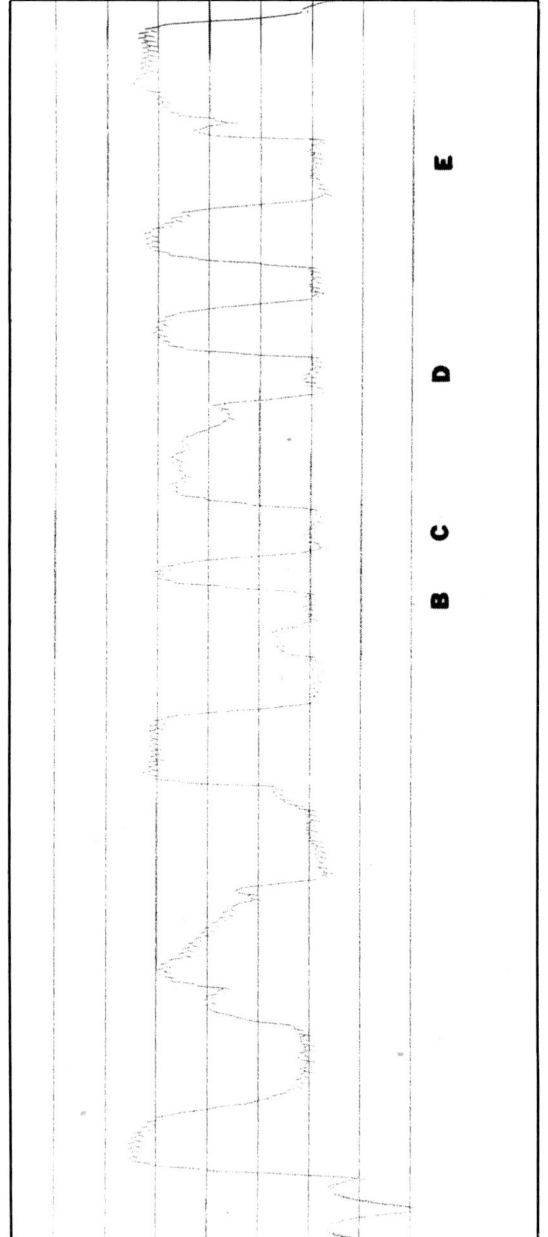

Figure 8-5 (top).

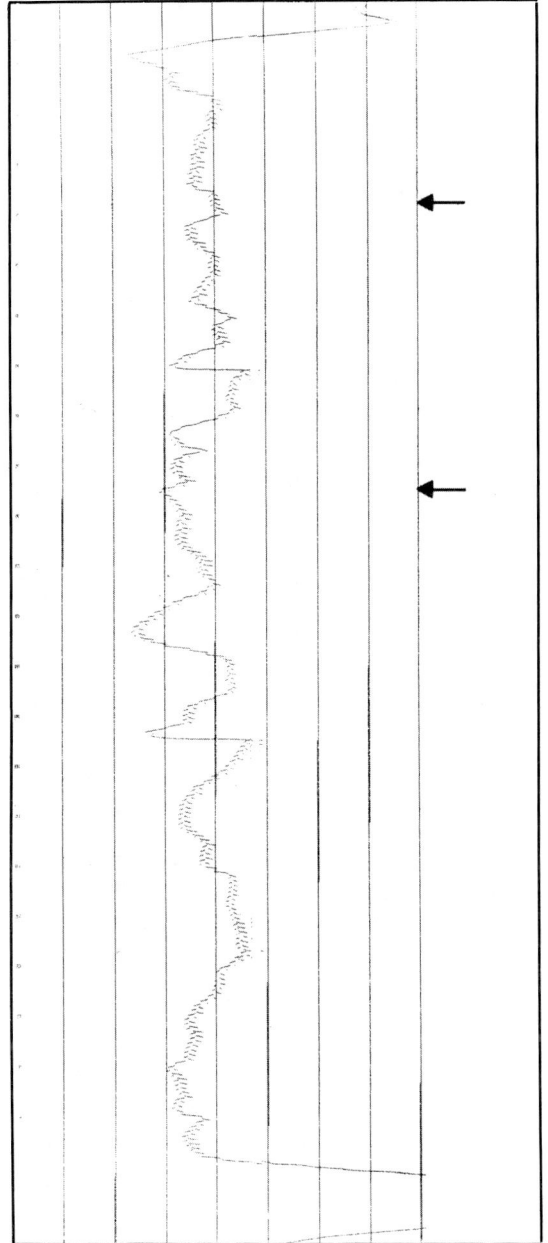

Figure 8-5 (bottom). Averaged amplitude displays of a good (top) and poor (bottom) artificial larynx speaker's production of "This suit needs to go to the cleaners." The amplitude displays were generated from the productions illustrated in Fig. 8-4. Features highlighted by letters or arrows are explained in the text. The distance between each horizontal line represents 6 dB.

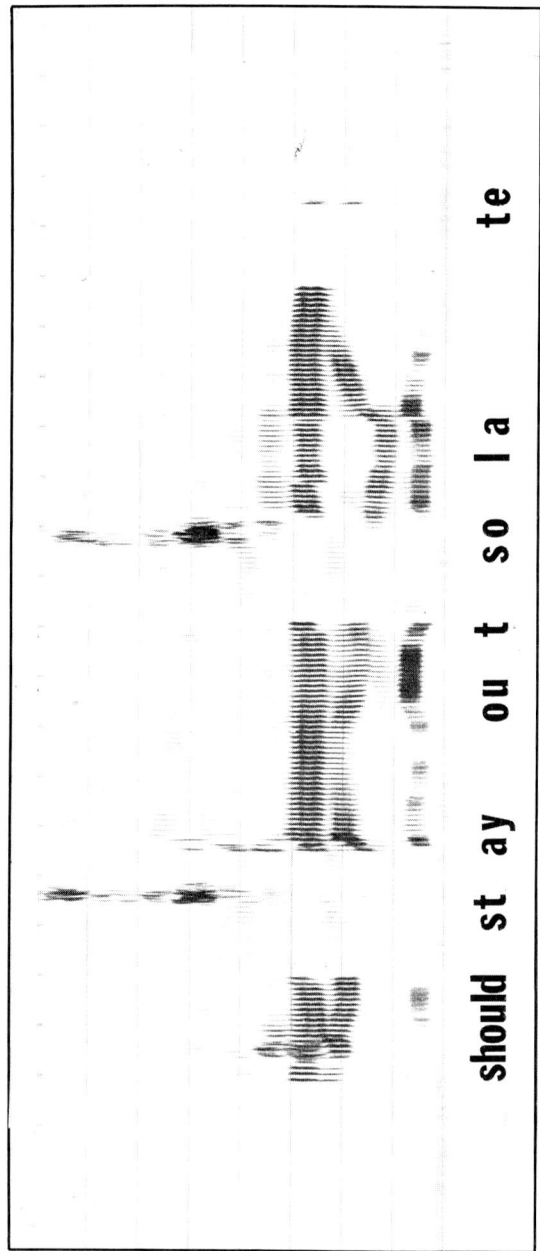

Figure 8-6 (top).

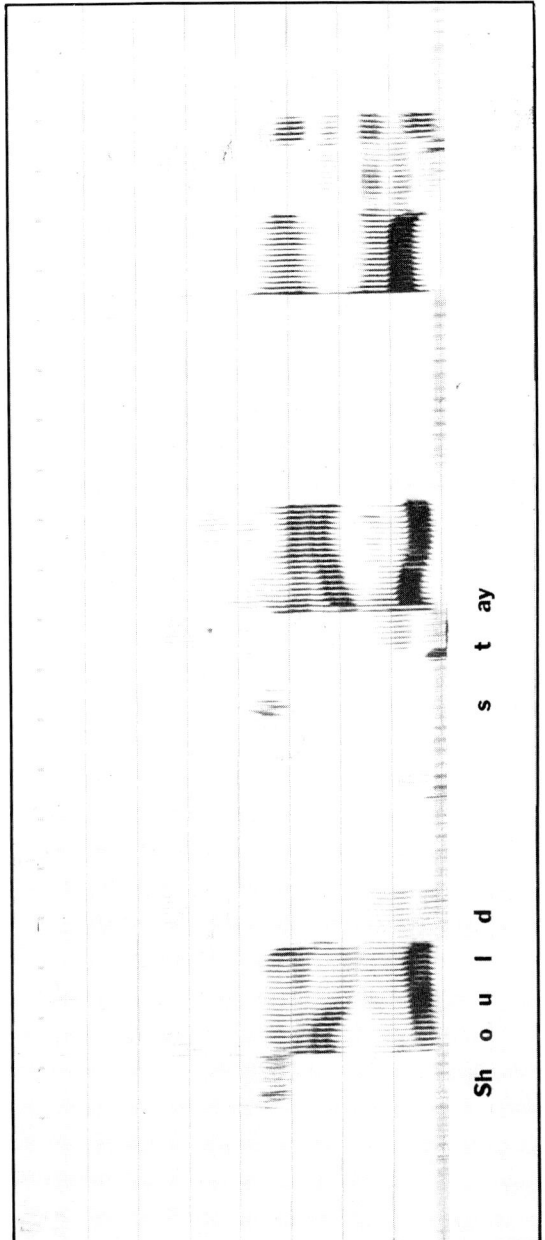

Figure 8-6 (bottom). Wide-band spectrograms of a good (top) and poor (bottom) artificial larynx speaker's production of "should stay out so late." The orthographic representations are spaced to approximate the appearance of the associated acoustic events.

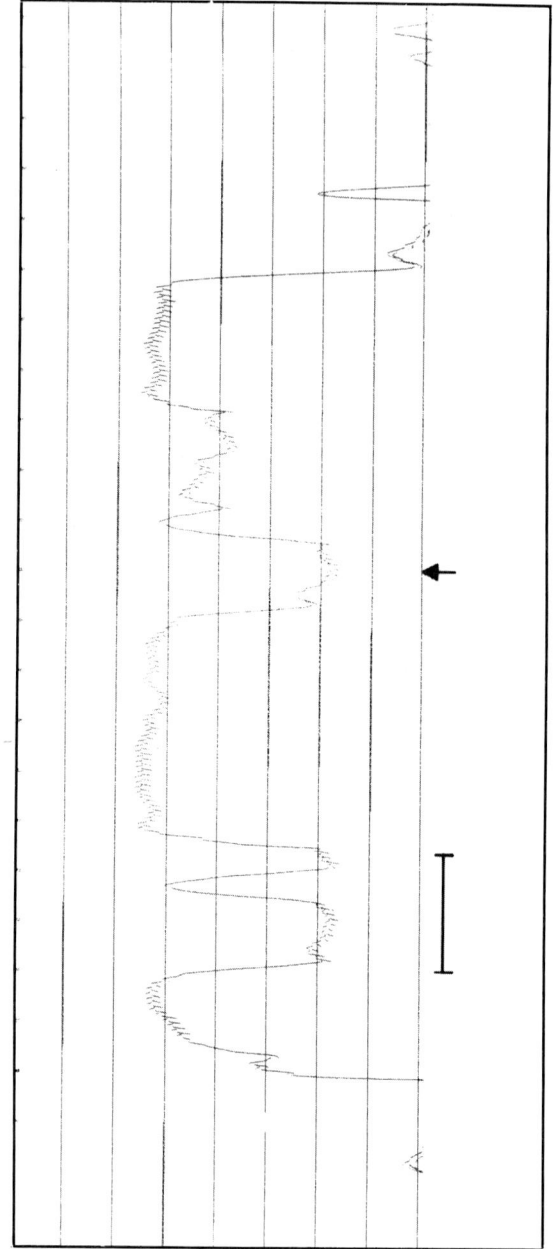

Figure 8-7 (top).

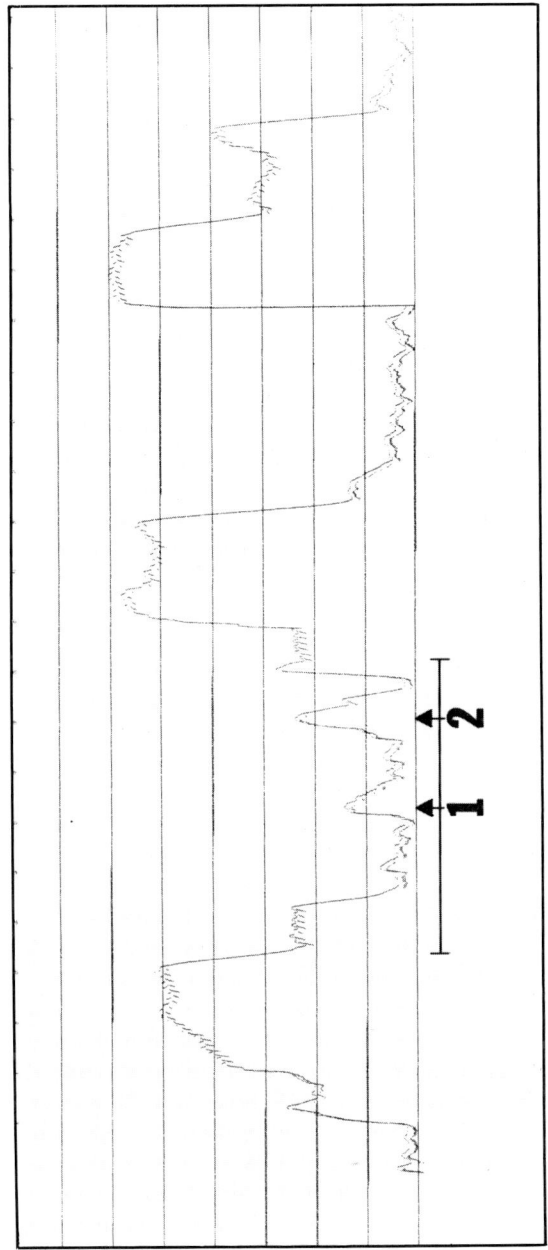

Figure 8-7 (bottom). Averaged amplitude displays of a good (top) and poor (bottom) artificial larynx speaker's production of "should stay out so late." The amplitude displays were generated from the productions illustrated in Fig. 8-6. Marked or numbered features are explained in the text. The difference between each horizontal line represents 6 dB.

fricative energy overlaid on the duty-cycle of the electronic larynx. Air flow and pressure measurements indicated similar differences. When these differences were not apparent, perceptual confusions resulted.

Isshiki and Tanabe recognized the inherent limitations in single-subject investigations, and were guarded in their conclusions about the mechanisms involved in producing the differences they observed. However, their methodology has great clinical significance for objectively measuring the speech of artificial larynx users and for ascertaining the need for appropriate rehabilitation.

CONCLUSIONS

Additional study is necessary to provide a complete description of artificial larynx speech. Perceptual ratings and laboratory instrumentation and methodologies are available for classifying artificial larynx users as poor, good, and superior speakers, as well as for specifying the distinguishing features of speech that results in these categorizations.

The data presented in this chapter represent a small beginning. Additional information must be gathered on larger populations of electronic larynx users. Further, superior speakers must be identified and used in subsequent investigations. The tendency to discourage the use of the artificial larynx perhaps is due to a lack of familiarity with superior practitioners of the available devices.

According to the data presented here, the parameters related to speaking proficiency are:

1. Rate of speech.
2. Intensity range.
3. Presence or absence of extraneous noises.
4. Number of pauses per sentence.

The articulation factors for speaking proficiency are primarily intensity variations appropriate for closure and/or release of stop-consonants (voiced and voiceless), and for the delineation of fricative energy. Frequency range was expected to be an important parameter for distinguishing between good and poor speakers; however, it was not significant. The restricted frequency ranges utilized by the two groups emphasized the mechanical, artificial sound of the electronic larynx, but appeared to have little effect on intelligibility or on listener judgments of speaking proficiency. Implications for therapy provided by these data will be discussed in Part E of Chapter 9.

REFERENCES

1. Bailey BJ: Vocal rehabilitation after total laryngectomy. Transcripts from: Pacific Coast Oto-Opthal Soc 55:77–84, 1974
2. Bailey BJ, Goode RL: New and projected procedures and devices for voice rehabilitation after total laryngectomy. Can J Otol 4:605–609, 1975
3. Putney FJ: Rehabilitation of the post-laryngectomized patient: Specific discussion of failures, advanced and difficult technical problems. Ann Otol Rhinol Laryngol 69:544–549, 1958
4. Goldstein LP, Rothman HB: Analysis of speech produced with an artificial larynx. Presented at the American Speech and Hearing Association Convention, Houston, Texas, 1976
5. Davis H, Silverman RS: Hearing and Deafness. New York, Holt, Rinehart and Winston, 1960
6. Curry ET, Snidecor JC: Physical measurement and pitch perception in esophageal speech. Laryngoscope 71:3–11, 1961
7. Shipp T: Frequency, duration and perceptual measures in relation to judgments of alaryngeal speech acceptability. J Speech Hear Res 10:417–427, 1967
8. Bennett A, Weinberg B: Acceptability ratings of normal, esophageal and artificial larynx speech. J Speech Hear Res 16:608–615, 1973
9. Isshiki N, Tanabe M: Acoustic and aerodynamic study of a superior electrolarynx speaker. Folia Phoniatr 24:65–76, 1972
10. Rothman HB, Goldstein LP: Analysis of speech produced with an artificial larynx. Presented at the American Speech and Hearing Association Convention, Houston, Texas, 1976

Section IV

TREATMENT & CONCLUSIONS

This section presents various treatment considerations and a composite of ideas concerning the clinical, academic, and research approach to treatment. This information should provide clinicians with a basis for developing their own treatment strategies.

The last chapter summarizes the authors' current attitudes concerning artificial larynx devices. We encourage the early use of an artificial larynx in the speech rehabilitation program. Finally, predictions are presented regarding the use of artificial larynges for total rehabilitation of laryngectomees.

9.
Approaches to Treatment

Rather than presenting a cookbook approach to treatment, each contributing author was asked to submit a philosophy of treatment, a current technique, or a case history. We think that the results are exciting. The benefits of having six presentations and ideas outweighs the occasional repetition and possible conflicts. The authors are presented in alphabetical order.

Part A

WILLIAM R. BERRY

I have some strong feelings about the total rehabilitation of laryngectomized individuals. However, because of the charge and scope of this text, I will present only a few ideas relative to the use of artificial larynx devices in treatment. Some of my thoughts apply to laryngectomee rehabilitation in general, reflecting my philosophy of treatment in which I try to balance the scientific method with pragmatic humanism.

Initiation of Treatment

The objective is to *get them talking as soon as possible*. The early stages of communication therapy can be critical to later success. It is important that you and your patient have a clear understanding of the term success. If success is esophageal speech at any cost, then you should make sure that your patient is fully aware of the price in terms of time and effort that he must pay to reach this goal. Information sharing and truthful, open communication are vital at the initiation of treatment.

This is not a time to be the stereotype of a used-car salesman or the flim-flam man. It is not your larynx that has been removed, and you have no right to impose your opinions unless you have solid evidence supporting one type of treatment over another. Initially the patient should be presented with all the information for and against available treatment approaches. Remember that the patient is a consumer of health care. The ethics of our profession should make us aware of our roles both as consumer advocates and as producers of quality treatment techniques. If a good salesman has a quality product to sell, he is not afraid of the informed consumer; only the con man shades his product from the light in his pursuit of self-interest. We have a good product to sell.

Without realizing it, many clinicians who espouse an open-minded attitude about artificial larynges bias their patients against them merely by the method of initiating treatment. They may carefully explain all of the positive and negative aspects associated with both esophageal speech and the various types of artificial larynx devices, and then initiate treatment by working exclusively on esophageal speech. The reasons include lack of training with artificial larynx devices, bias, or unanalyzed clinical habits. Whatever the cause, the result may be a feeling of failure by the laryngectomee if he happens to be one of many who either develop poor esophageal speech or are unable to acquire it at all.

A combined approach at the outset of treatment can prevent later feelings of inadequacy on the part of the patient who may not be able to develop esophageal speech. There simply are no convincing data to support the view that issuing artificial devices early in treatment will impede the development of esophageal speech. However, we have all heard the argument that an artificial larynx is a crutch.

If this is the case, and the patient chooses to walk with a crutch after knowing all the facts, then so be it! Our job is to make sure that the patient receives all the information he needs to make a decision, and then to help him talk as well as possible. By letting the patient try a number of different artificial larynges early in treatment, and by also letting him have an opportunity to develop esophageal sound, the clinician conveys the attitude that serviceable, intelligible speech is important, not the type of alaryngeal speech. It is likely that speech recovery would be facilitated if the patient could develop this attitude. It is a principle of behavioral modification to start with easy tasks first and then to work toward more difficult ones. Few would deny that it is easier to develop intelligible speech with an artificial larynx than with esophageal speech.

APPROACHES TO TREATMENT

Treatment Progression

With this behavioral modification principle in mind, I believe that early treatment should emphasize—but not sell—artificial larynges. A reasonable formula might be 75 percent treatment time with alaryngeal devices and 25 percent treatment time with esophageal speech. If the proper device (intraoral, neck type, pneumatic) can be selected early, the patient will begin to interact verbally with the world. The foundation will have been laid for more sophisticated and difficult verbalization tasks. As treatment proceeds, the formula can be shifted by mutual consent until, only a few weeks after the initiation of treatment, the patient spends equal time on both esophageal speech and the artificial larynx of choice.

This is especially important if the therapist is a hospital clinician or in private practice. Many times laryngectomees cannot be treated by speech pathologists after being discharged from the hospital; due to geographic distance, they are unable to return for treatment or cannot be referred to another clinician. If the combined approach is utilized early in treatment, it becomes possible for the patient to be speaking with an artificial larynx device at the time of hospital discharge, possibly even well enough to be understood over the telephone. The combined therapy then can proceed by telephone therapy or Tel-Communication[1] and the patient is not left to adapt, or to attempt to relearn verbal communication, on his own.

Later, if the patient begins to progress in esophageal speech to a phrase-length output, the time formula should shift to meet the pace of improvement. However, I do not recommend that the device be omitted from treatment unless the *patient* decides that he does not want to use it any more. Often, patients who have learned serviceable esophageal speech discover that there are times when their speech breaks down or is not intelligible. In these instances, patients who know how to use an artificial larynx will have a positive attitude and will not hesitate to use the device.

I believe that part of the treatment should continue to refine the patient's artificial larynx speech even after he has developed some esophageal speech, in order to build a more positive attitude toward the device. I have unfortunately encountered clinicians who decided that their patients had "arrived" with an artificial larynx when speech was intelligible, and thereafter encouraged their patients to concentrate on esophageal speech all of the time. When the clinician terminates instruction with the artificial larynx, the laryngectomee must assume that his progress with the device has reached a plateau. Complaints that we often hear about the mechanical quality of artificial larynx devices may be the result of poor follow-up and training in the prosodic refinements of speech with these devices. The laryngectomee will be continually encouraged to use his artificial larynx if a small percentage of time for prosodic refinement drills is retained during the later stages of treatment.

Summary

The following statements summarize my beliefs concerning the use of artificial larynx devices for laryngectomee rehabilitation.

1. Let the patient decide whether he wants to learn esophageal speech or to use an artificial larynx after receiving all the pertinent information he needs to make that decision.
2. Have a supply of various types of alaryngeal devices available, plus audio or video tapes demonstrating their use, to maximize the opportunity for the patient to find a device that he can utilize effectively.
3. Arrange for visitations from a laryngectomee who utilizes both esophageal speech and an artificial larynx device proficiently, so that the patient will not become biased.
4. Use a combined approach from the outset of treatment, teaching both esophageal speech and the use of the artificial larynx of choice.
5. Make sure that the entire rehabilitation team (that is, surgeon, nurse, social worker, physical therapist, family members) is well informed about artificial larynx devices.
6. Try to refine the patient's use of his device especially with regard to prosodic speech dimensions, as long as communication treatment continues.
7. Promote research projects that will yield more information comparing intelligibility and acceptability of esophageal speech with various types of artificial larynx devices.

REFERENCE

1. Vaughn G: Tel-communicology: Health-care delivery systems for persons with communicative disorder. ASMA J 18:13–17, 1976

Part B

ERIC D. BLOM

Instruction in the use of an artificial larynx requires a step-by-step systematic approach not unlike that utilized in the acquisition of esophageal speech. My approach consists chiefly of a set of fundamental skill-building strategies, followed by a series of instructional units designed to achieve highly profi-

APPROACHES TO TREATMENT

cient communication with an artificial larynx. Fundamental skills consist of effective instrument placement and accurate timing of voice-source activation and termination. Refinement exercises focus on articulation, phrasing, rate, inflection, and stress. These skills should be mastered in the order that they will be discussed here.

Preliminaries to Instruction

Initiation of artificial larynx speech training frequently must be preceded by making minor adjustments to the commercial artificial larynx in order to make it "fit" the individual user. Pitch and loudness characteristics of electronic mouth-type and neck-type instruments should be adjusted and pre-set to provide the most appropriate voice. Excessive extraneous noise radiating from the head of some neck-type electronic larynges (for example, Western Electric No. 5) can be reduced by packing foam rubber in and around the space occupied by the vibrator. Goode[1] suggests that the problem of saliva blockage in the mouth-tube of electronic mouth-type instruments can be eliminated by loosely covering the open end of the tube with a .005 inch-thick piece of Silastic.

Adjustments to the stoma coupling attachment, the sound-producing mechanism, and the mouth tube of pneumatic devices are almost always mandatory in order to fit the instrument to the individual user. Tracheostoma depth, angle, and location frequently make it difficult to achieve an airtight seal easily with the standard stoma cover provided with the instrument. In these instances, the standard stoma coupling must either be modified or replaced. For example, the rubber stoma cup provided with the Tokyo artificial larynx can be turned inside out to fit into the rim of the stoma rather than over it. Items that can be used to replace the standard stoma cover and make an airtight seal include the flexible flanged end of a Bardex fistula tube, a small flexible rubber shower head, or other innovative items. A custom-made coupling also may be fabricated by a maxillo-facial prosthodontist at minimal expense. Use of all nonstandard stoma cover adaptations should have medical approval prior to routine application.

Most pneumatic artificial larynges have an adjustable vibrating mechanism that consists of either a rubber membrane or a plastic reed. It is necessary to experimentally adjust the length, width, and tension of these vibrators to achieve an easily activated voice source that provides appropriate pitch and loudness variability. Once this "tuning" has been accomplished, the user must learn to achieve vocal flexibility by changing pulmonary air flow and pressure. Mouth-tube length and shape also must be adjusted to accommodate easy and unobtrusive use of the pneumatic artificial larynx. The tube should be cut to a length so that $\frac{3}{4}$-inch of it can be inserted in the mouth without an excessive amount left over. Permanent tube curvature, angle, and rigidity can easily be achieved by inserting a 5-inch piece of stainless steel wire inside the tube to maintain proper configuration.

Fundamental Skills

PLACEMENT

Effective placement is one of the most fundamental skills to be mastered with an artificial larynx. The user must learn to couple the instrument to his vocal tract to achieve maximum sound transfer. With electronic neck-type instruments, the point of coupling is between the vibratory head of the instrument and a suitable soft spot in the cervical neck tissue. Contact must be relatively firm and flush to eliminate leakage of sound. Once the optimal contact point has been identified, it can be marked with tape or magic marker to facilitate accurate placement.

The mouth tube of an electronic mouth-type instrument should be placed along the inner lateral surface of the upper first and second molar, thereby avoiding blockage by saliva and by the skin lining of the cheek. The tube should enter from the corner of the mouth and be inserted about $\frac{3}{4}$-inch. This manner of placement minimizes the tube's interference with tongue and lip articulation.

Pneumatic artificial larynges require what amounts to double placement, since the instrument must be coupled both into the mouth and over the stoma. The user should be taught first to insert the tube in his mouth, and then to cover the stoma. Although some users can achieve a good airtight stoma seal without removing their knit stoma cover, others find it necessary to flip this knit cover to one side before coupling the pneumatic device to the stoma.

Placement drills for all types of artificial larynges consist of exercises first to achieve accurate placement, and then to achieve rapid accurate placement. Drills should initially be done in front of a mirror. The objective is 100 percent accurate placement in 0.5 seconds or less. In all cases the user should be taught to hold the artificial larynx in his nondominant hand and to keep his dominant hand free.

TIMING

Accurate onset and termination of voicing, simultaneous with the corresponding speech utterance, is a necessary skill for using an artificial larynx effectively. Most users have a tendency to activate their device after they have started to talk, or to prematurely terminate voicing before the end of the utterance. The user should practice producing single words, phrases, paragraphs, and conversational speech over a tape recorder in order to master accurate timing of voicing. Accuracy should be monitored and practice continued until 100 percent success is achieved.

ARTICULATION

Speech articulation is significantly altered after laryngectomy and requires considerable attention if normal or near normal intelligibility is to be achieved. Prior to initiation of speech training, the clinician should review the operative report and conduct an oral peripheral speech mechanism examination to determine potential structural, motor, or sensory deficits.

Only minimal instruction is generally required to achieve precise articulation of vowels, unless there are gross alterations to the articulatory mechanism. Conversely, extensive training is almost always necessary to produce accurate consonants. The artificial larynx user must learn to compensate for his altered ability to generate plosive and fricative noise, as well as accurate voicing features, both of which signal perceptually important contrasts between cognate phoneme pairs in the English language.

I agree with Isshiki[2] that artificial larynx users may be better able to produce significant contrast between cognates—such as /p/ and /b/ or /s/ and /z/—by focusing on aerodynamic features rather than by trying to learn to incorporate the voice/voiceless distinction. That is, the user should learn to produce exaggerated plosive or fricative noise as the distinguishing feature of voiceless consonants. This noise must be significant enough to override any inappropriately timed voicing that may inadvertently be heard during production of voiceless consonants. Since the pulmonary airstream no longer participates in speech production except when a pneumatic artificial larynx is used, the user must learn to generate high intra-oral–pharyngeal air pressure with residual air in his mouth. Voiced consonants should be produced with voicing and negligible plosive or fricative noise.

PHRASING AND RATE

Normalization of phrasing and rate of speech with an artificial larynx can be achieved easily by following the exercises described by Fairbanks.[3] In almost all cases only a brief amount of time must be spent in these areas. The user needs to be made aware of acceptable rate and phrasing, and to be provided with the opportunity to tape-record his practice exercises.

INFLECTION AND STRESS

Incorporation of inflection and stress into artificial larynx speech is limited by the type of instrument being used, which is unfortunate when the common observation made by listeners is that "artificial larynx speech sounds monotonous." With the exception of the Western Electric No. 5 artificial larynx and pneumatic instruments, pitch and loudness characteristics are pre-set. With the Western Electric No. 5, pitch can be varied over half an octave during speech by changing the degree to which the thumb-operated control knob is depressed. Thumb control of linguistically correct pitch variability during running speech represents a challenging task; and a diligent attempt to teach this skill should be made with all users who demonstrate reasonable potential. Fairbanks[3] provides excellent inflection drill exercises.

Linguistically appropriate pitch and loudness variability with pneumatic artificial larynges is a natural and easily obtainable skill, chiefly because voicing with these instruments is aerodynamically dictated. The user must learn that increases and decreases in breath pressure, which are similar to those used when producing voice with a normal larynx, result in loudness and pitch variability with the pneumatic artificial larynx. Practice with the inflection and stress drill exercises in Fairbanks[3] usually results in rapid attainment of these skills.

REFERENCES

1. Goode RL: Artificial laryngeal devices in post-laryngectomy rehabilitation. Laryngoscope 85:677–689, 1975
2. Isshiki N, Tanabe M: Acoustic and aerodynamic study of a superior electrolarynx speaker. Folia Phoniatr 24:65–76, 1972
3. Fairbanks G: Voice and Articulation Drillbook. New York, Harper, 1959

Part C

MARSHALL J. DUGUAY

I have had the opportunity to work in a variety of professional employment settings, including public schools, a hospital clinic, a community hearing and speech center, private practice, and a college program. This statement is meant neither as an indictment nor as a call for applause. It is intended to remind the reader that I am particularly cognizant of programmatic constraints. It is possible to hold lofty ideals only to find their implementation impossible. Consequently, the ideal approach to the use of the artificial larynx may have to be modified in order to achieve a reasonable goal.

APPROACHES TO TREATMENT

Selection of Devices

Clearly, as I stated in Chapter 1, I believe in the concurrent teaching of esophageal and artificial larynx speech. This means that the clinician needs to have a *selection* of devices available to try with a patient in order to best serve his individual needs. There is no ideal instrument. Characteristics of an instrument and the needs of a patient greatly vary. If funds are available to purchase one of each instrument, the problem is solved. If funds are not available, writing to each company to ask for a demonstration device is an avenue to explore. Many times a service group such as the Sertoma Club, Lions, or Rotary will be willing to purchase a device for a lending bank. The term "lending bank" is used for I believe that each patient, whenever possible, should procure his own device—either with private funds or through state, federal, or third-party agencies. When a person has his own device, the device he borrowed can be made available for others. Sometimes a local Laryngectomee Club will prove helpful by creating a collection of devices for loan. Many times families will donate the artificial larynx of a deceased laryngectomee to a training program, especially if it is a clinical program that is housed in a hospital or university environment. The greater the variety of devices available, the more likely that the patient can be furnished with the appropriate device.

Several years ago I worked in a situation where funds were not readily available except to purchase only one or two devices. I therefore set up a study[1] to determine if there were differences in intelligibility between seven different devices. Phonetically-balanced word lists were used as the basis for intelligibility ratings, and both sophisticated and naive listeners scored the speakers. The devices compared were: Western Electric No. 5 (revised model with the tapered head), Western Electric No. 5 (original model with the flat head), Aurex, Cooper-Rand, Dutch DSP 8, Western Electric pneumatic device, and the Tait Oral Vibrator. With the exception of the Tait Oral Vibrator,[2] possibly because of a poor fitting in the patient's mouth, there were no statistically significant differences in intelligibility among the devices. I suspect that this finding still applies for all commercially available devices. However, there were noticeable differences in the perceived quality. Since communication necessitates a receiver as well as a sender, quality is an important consideration. You can appreciate this quality factor if you have listened to the audio tape that accompanies this text. Therefore the general factors of availability, price, and quality will influence the selection of a device for a patient.

There is one other general aspect that needs to be considered: cosmesis. In my opinion the pneumatic devices, though certainly very pleasing in quality, are too noticeable and attention-drawing. They also require direct access to the stoma. For these two reasons, some patients may elect not to try a pneumatic device. Others are perfectly satisfied with this type.

Even in this brief discussion the subjective aspects of selecting an artificial larynx become apparent. In order to minimize subjectivity, it can be very helpful to tape-record the same material using several different devices. This experience is especially helpful for the patient in overcoming any bias that he may have because he hears himself differently than others hear him. He needs to realize that the way he sounds on tape is the way he is heard by the listener. We constantly must remind ourselves that our subjective judgments are secondary to those of the patient and should not be imposed on him. His satisfaction, not ours, is the goal. Usually, however, there is close agreement.

Once we have considered availability, cost, quality, and cosmesis in the choice of a device, we still have much to do in helping a patient learn to use it effectively.

NECK-TYPE DEVICES

I make it a point to teach the patient to use the device by holding it in his nondominant hand. This allows him use of his preferred hand for other activities. For example, he can cradle the telephone between his head and shoulder, activate the device with his nondominant hand, and still be able to write telephone messages.

The principle in using the neck-type device is to transfer maximum sound into the oral cavity where it can be articulated into meaningful speech. Therefore, placement of the device becomes a critical issue.

A clinical phenomena that can prove extremely frustrating is the patient whose placement appears satisfactory, yet who does not seem to have sound available in his oral cavity. Moving the device laterally, medially, or in any other direction does not help. The problem is that the sound does not enter the oral cavity because the patient is carrying his tongue in a high and retracted position. The device, held to the neck area, allows the sound to enter the pharynx, where it becomes trapped; the retracted tongue seals off the oral cavity, disallowing sound transmission into the oral area.

Once identified, the problem can be corrected easily. Two of my favorite techniques are:

1. Instruct the patient to activate the electronic larynx and then to *talk* on inhalation. The sound will no longer be sealed in the pharynx, since the tongue drops and flattens during the inhalation part of the respiratory cycle to permit maximum air flow to the lungs. The patient hears an appropriate acoustic target which he can attempt to copy on the exhalation part of the respiratory cycle.

APPROACHES TO TREATMENT

2. Have the patient stick his tongue out as far as possible, activate the device, and talk (count, days of the week, etc.) even with the resulting lack of intelligibility. The anterior tongue position prevents humping and retraction, allows entry of sound into the oral cavity, and furnishes a target for the patient to model by using graduated increments of tongue movement back into a normal position within the oral cavity.

This is not an especially common problem, but it can be vexing when confronted for the first time. Since it is an acoustic problem, the reader can hear an example of the problem and a demonstration of the techniques for solving it on the tape accompanying the text (Side I, Demonstration A).

Correct placement of the electronic larynx is a very individualized procedure. The clinician will want to avoid a neck area that presents with edema or cicatricial tissue. Care should be taken not to place the vibrator over a suture line, since the line might break the tight seal necessary for maximum sound introduction. If possible, both sides of the neck, midline, and submental areas should be tried to find the area permitting greatest sound transmission. When only limited areas are available because of a patient's small structure or surgical violation, the size of head on the device becomes important; it is sometimes helpful to explore areas for placement with a smaller-headed device. Once the best spot is located, other instruments can be applied to that spot.

The patient who wears a hearing aid may prove somewhat of a problem. He probably will be better able to monitor his speech output if the device can be held on the contralateral side from the hearing aid receiver. The amplified buzz may result in a masking noise for his speech output monitoring as well as cause annoyance or discomfort, and he may therefore reject the instrument.

After the correct spot is identified, some patients experience difficulty in relocating and returning their device to it. Others may fail to keep a flush contact between the device and the area. The electronic larynx must be held firm and flush to the spot or the generated sound will leak into the environment rather than enter the pharyngeal-oral region where it belongs. Visualizing the spot and practicing before a mirror may be all that is necessary for some patients. Others who still have a problem returning the device to the correct site, and many honestly do, will need a more direct approach. The clinician can take a magic marker or a felt tip pen and actually outline or "X" the spot. Then, using this visual clue in front of a mirror, they can practice hitting the spot until a tactile and motor response is established. A small piece of tape can be fixed to the area if practice is done without a mirror.

Treatment must include work on starting and stopping the device appropriately. The tendency for some patients is simply to activate the instrument and keep talking through to completion of the message unit. This makes speech very mechanical and monotonous. The patient needs to work on phrasing. As one patient so aptly stated, "I need to remember to talk with commas and periods." Listen critically to be sure that the instrument stays activated to the very end of the utterance. And if the utterance ends with an unvoiced consonant, make sure that the device is stopped appropriately so that, for example, "cat" does not become "cata" with an intruded schwa. Drills and exercises can be devised to practice these goals.

Instruction in the use of the Western Electric No. 5 should include work on varying pitch so that the supra-segmental cues enhance the message as well as combat the inherent monotonous tone of the electronic larynx. On all other electronic devices, the dials controlling frequency as well as intensity are fixed in a way that renders access to them nearly impossible during running speech.

CONCLUDING REMARKS

Let us focus on two general concepts which are relevant for all devices. First, many electronic devices contain dials to adjust frequency and intensity of sound. Some patients inadvertently manipulate these dials as they place or remove the device from a pocket or purse. To prevent this from occurring, a piece of tape can be placed over the dials after the best settings have been determined.

Second, it seems to me that as clinicians we often fail to take reality testing into account. We rarely leave the treatment room to see how the laryngectomee uses his artificial larynx device in the real world. We should not assume that because he uses the device well with us in therapy, he uses it equally as well in a store, bank, or restaurant. He may be embarrassed or reluctant to use it with strangers or in a particular situation. Perhaps the anxiety and tension generated by new experiences cause him to place the device on a less than perfect spot. Or perhaps someone with a hearing impairment responds inappropriately. He may erroneously believe that he is at fault rather than the listener. Unless the clinician knows exactly what happened, he can neither counsel adequately nor devise therapy strategies to alleviate the problem. Therefore, be sure to build real-life experiences into the regular therapy sessions, to assist the laryngectomee in using his artificial larynx in the most effective way.

Daniel Webster is reported to have said, "If all my possessions were taken from me with one exception, I would choose to keep the power of speech, for with it I would soon regain all the rest." Our laryngectomee patients may need to be reminded that they have not lost their power of speech. It is not lost, but merely different, and it is our differences that make us interesting human beings.

REFERENCES

1. Duguay MJ: Intelligibility ratings of seven different artificial larynges—A pilot investigation. Presented at the American Speech and Hearing Association Convention, Denver, Colorado, 1967
2. Tait RV: The oral vibrator. Brit Dent J 106:336–340, 1959

Part D

LEWIS P. GOLDSTEIN

In the past few years, I have come to realize as a result of clinical experience and research that procedures for teaching the proper use of an artificial larynx are complex. The notion that all the clinician has to do is provide a laryngectomee with an artificial larynx for him to speak proficiently is the same as simply telling the stutterer to speak normally. Each laryngectomee presents different problems. However, certain broad concepts must be understood by all laryngectomees using an artificial larynx, including

1. Acceptance;
2. Consistency;
3. Intelligibility.

Acceptance

Acceptance of an artificial larynx by the laryngectomee is highly dependent upon the clinician. If the clinician is not completely convinced that the artificial larynx has an important role in alaryngeal rehabilitation, the laryngectomee will undoubtedly be reluctant to use the instrument. It is hoped that by now most, if not all, clinicians' attitudes toward the artificial larynx have become one of complete acceptance.

One way that positive attitudes can be conveyed to the laryngectomee is by introducing him to other laryngectomees who use an artificial larynx. Perhaps the clinician too can use an artificial larynx. The actual giving of the device can also convey many hidden meanings. Handing the laryngectomee a box and having him open it to find a device which further must be taken apart, fitted with batteries, and reassembled presents a picture of the artificial larynx as cumbersome, bothersome, and mechanically complicated. In contrast, presenting the laryngectomee with a device (minus the box) that is already in working order indicates that it is ready to be used and does not have to be played with. The mechanical process can be explained in subsequent sessions. If he is not given the original box, the laryngectomee is more likely to find another place to store the device, perhaps in a convenient pocket, on a string around his neck, or on his belt—as many calculators or eyeglasses are placed.

Finally, to aid in naturalness and therefore in acceptance of the artificial larynx, it is recommended that the device be used with the nondominant hand. This allows the dominant hand to be free for writing, drinking, eating, and gesturing. By having his dominant hand free, the laryngectomee is more likely to hold the device for longer periods of time and to use the artificial larynx for casual remarks.

Consistency-of-Placement Program

Consistency in the placement of the artificial larynx is one of the most important factors leading to proficient speech. It is usually the first feature to be worked on and also the most easily programmed.

1. Obtain the ideal neck placement through trial and error. Mark the area with a small piece of tape.
2. With the device held in place by the laryngectomee, first have him produce a sound with correct placement; then have him produce a poor sound caused by improper placement or coupling. Discuss and compare the perceptual differences.
3. Have the laryngectomee consistently produce a series of sounds with the device correctly placed. This should be done in front of a mirror and with the aid of a small piece of tape marking the area of ideal neck placement.
4. Have the laryngectomee produce a series of sounds, one immediately after another, using correct placement. However, he must remove the device from his neck after each sound. This is also to be done in front of a mirror and with the aid of the tape as a marker.
5. Finally, have the laryngectomee produce a series of good sounds without the aid of the tape marker and/or the mirror.

A criteria of 90 percent correct placement over three days for steps 3, 4, and 5 should be set. Performance should be graphed so that improvement can be seen easily.

When the therapist stresses consistency of correct placement, the laryngectomee gains confidence that he is using the artificial larynx correctly.

Better listener acceptance will be achieved as the laryngectomee learns to avoid extraneous noises produced by poor coupling.

Intelligibility

Intelligibility is the most important factor in artificial larynx speech. Accepting the device and achieving excellent consistency of placement are useless if the laryngectomee cannot produce intelligible speech. Only a speech disorder that existed prior to surgery or extensive surgery involving the articulators should preclude the acquisition of intelligible speech. Unfortunately, there is a tendency among clinicians and laryngectomees to slow down the rate of speech and to over-articulate when using a device. This tendency decreases intelligibility by distorting the inherent rhythms of language: it also increases the mechanical and artificial aspects of speech. Direct treatment is usually needed in two areas.

First, the laryngectomee must learn to control the activation mechanism. He should be able to turn the sound on and off quickly. He needs to develop a sense for how long the sound can be kept on before it becomes overpowering and annoying to the listener. At the same time, constant, rhythmic on–off manipulations also are distracting. Examples can be heard on the accompanying cassette (Side II, Demonstration B). As the laryngectomee learns to control the activation mechanism, a normal rate of speech should be emphasized. Combining activation of the on–off switch with normal phrasing and rate is a very useful exercise.

Second, the laryngectomee must learn to distinguish between voiced and voiceless sounds. Once he has gained complete control of the activation mechanism, he should employ this ability into distinguishing between paired words. With good feedback and practice, the laryngectomee should be able to master this task. A sample of an individual practicing paired words is on the cassette (Side II, Demonstration C).

In order to integrate acceptability, consistency, and intelligibility of artificial larynx speech, general conversation and *normal* feedback should be stressed. It is suggested by normal feedback that when the laryngectomee's reply is not understood the clinician should respond with "Excuse me," "I beg your pardon," or "Did you say . . . or . . . ." This type of response gives the laryngectomee practice in deciding what his error is and how to correct it; it also trains him to use his environment to maintain and improve his speech.

Part E

HOWARD B. ROTHMAN

This section reflects an experimentalist point of view relative to some of the problems encountered by laryngectomees using an artificial larynx. These opinions are not based on preconceived clinical techniques, but on laboratory-type measurements of signal output. My intent is to add a scientific perspective to the clinical approach.

In my opinion, the following considerations are of primary importance when planning or initiating a rehabilitation program that involves the use of an electronic larynx.

1. Most laryngectomees were normal speakers and would still be normal speakers for their age group if it were not for surgical removal of the larynx.
2. Clinical observations over a number of years have demonstrated that a functional articulatory mechanism is retained by laryngectomees after surgery. Support for these observations, which are restricted to users of electronic larynges, can be found in statements by Stetson,[1] Kallen,[2] and Morton.[3] Their statements support the conclusion that problems affecting speech are related more to aerodynamics than to articulation.

Goals for treatment of many speech disorders are often based on various models, such as the average talker for a particular age group, dialectal area, or perhaps the clinician. However, there are few models for the laryngectomee who wants to utilize an electronic larynx. In Chapter 8 I discussed research involving artificial larynx users categorized as good and poor speakers, and I referred to a study by Isshiki and Tanabe[4] which utilized a superior electronic larynx speaker. Although no criteria were provided for the selection of the superior speaker, it can be surmised from the data why the selection was made: a good or superior electronic larynx user should be able to produce intelligible speech. In part, this means making voiced/voiceless distinctions—for example, contrasting /b/ and /p/, and /s/ and /z/—which involves more than producing a series of discrete, differentiated "clean" signals.

Speech is more than a series of discrete and invariant acoustic events; it is a dynamic and continuously varying acoustic event that can be perceived because of many different factors, such as knowledge of the language, expectations, and facial expressions. In addition, the listener most likely produces similar varying acoustic events in the same way as the speaker. Intelligibility is degraded if a speaker distorts the varying acoustic events called speech by altering the articulatory dynamics or the rhythms of the language.

Further, perception in oral communication is often enhanced by a hierarchy of acoustic cues. Some of these acoustic cues may be present as part of the signal before, during, and even after a particular speech sound. Both the variety and the temporal sequencing of the acoustic cues result in perceptual efficiency, which reduces the ambiguity that can often occur when competing signals are in the environment. For example, the acoustic parameters which serve as important cues for identifying a stop consonant in a vowel-consonant-vowel (that is, intervocalic) environment are:

1. The degree, extent, and rate of the formant transition to the consonant. Transitions represent articulatory movement from (or to) the place of consonant production to (or from) the position of the adjacent vowel.
2. Duration of the silent interval; that is, the stop phase. The closure duration for a voiced intervocalic stop tends to be shorter than for a voiceless one.
3. Presence of absence of voicing during the silent interval.
4. Voice onset time.
5. Duration of the noise burst, which may follow the release from the silent interval.
6. Spectral characteristic of the noise burst.
7. The vowel that precedes a voiced intervocalic stop tending to be longer than the same vowel before a voiceless stop.
8. The degree, extent, and rate of the formant transition to the following vowel.[5,6]

The multiplicity of cues and the parallel delivery of information provide a degree of redundancy. That is, a single acoustic segment carries information simultaneously about preceding and successive segments. This phenomenon is called coarticulation, and it partly functions to optimize listener ability to identify a phoneme or sequence of phonemes in difficult situations—such as a noisy environment or when large amounts of information must be processed quickly.[7] In an ideal listening (perceptual processing) situation, fewer of the available cues may suffice for optimal perception.

The preceding discussion is necessary. Too often the clinician is confronted with statements suggesting the introduction of acoustic and temporal distortions. One such suggestion is that proper use of an electronic larynx is dependent on speaking slowly, elongating vowels and syllables, overemphasizing certain sounds, and using a staccato-like rhythm based on syllabic units. There are several problems with this approach to treatment. First, it can introduce acoustic and temporal distortion to the speech production process and the parameters serving as perceptual cues may be obscured or modified. Second, an emotionally and physically traumatized individual with a functional articulatory system and an habituated speech pattern of perhaps forty-plus years is being requested to change that pattern. Third, artificiality due to the very nature of the electronic larynx is presently unavoidable and difficult to accept by both speaker and listener. Yet many approaches to treatment seem geared toward adding an additional artificial constraint to the development of intelligible speech.

The problem is that the source of voicing and air flow/pressure has been altered. Means of controlling the voicing mechanism and for developing adequate buccal pressure should be the primary concern of treatment. Therefore, particular care is necessary when helping a laryngectomee choose an artificial larynx. For example, a person who habitually (presurgically) spoke without much inflection may not be an ideal candidate for a device with a varying pitch control; or an individual with osteo or rheumatoid arthritis may not have the digital dexterity necessary to utilize a pitch control.

After an artificial larynx has been chosen and proper placement and coupling have been established, training for speech proficiency can begin by stressing (a) pitch and intensity variation; and (b) use of buccal air.

Pitch and Intensity Variation

Slight variations in pitch can be achieved even with electronic larynges that lack a variable frequency control. The vibrating disc or membrane which couples to the neck tissues is often driven by mechanical action involving a plunger. Coupling pressure can be varied by increasing or decreasing the pressure of the device on the neck, which causes a change in the frequency of vibration, and therefore of perceived pitch. Intensity varies in much the same way because of the dampening effect of increased coupling pressure on the movement of the plunger and vibrating disc (see Chapter 8).

Use of Buccal Air

In the laryngectomee, air no longer travels from the lungs through the trachea and into the oral cavity. Therefore other means for increasing air pressure and air flow are necessary. Buccal air should be used effectively by the laryngectomee in the production of stops, fricatives, and affricates. Production of initial stops can be practiced along with coordinating activation of the larynx.

The easiest way to begin is by producing an initial voiced-stop consonant. All one has to do in this case is activate the artificial larynx and open the mouth to talk. For an initial voiceless stop, the mouth should be opened before the artificial larynx is activated in order to produce some aspiration.

APPROACHES TO TREATMENT

Intervocalic plosives do not require deactivation of the artificial larynx or a pause. Habitual coupling pressure can be increased to attenuate the electronic larynx sound slightly at the same moment that closure occurs preceding the stop-release. The voiced/voiceless distinction can be made by varying the intensity of the release of buccal air, or by increasing the length of time that the artificial larynx sound is attenuated. Intervocalic fricatives also can be differentiated by varying the sharpness of the fricative noise.

Figure 9-1 is a spectrogram and amplitude display of a superior electronic speaker saying, "Do you think she should stay out so late?" The areas above the arrows indicate that attenuation of the electronic larynx buzz is possible in order to differentiate stop consonants. Frication is indicated, and it is produced by use of buccal air. It is audible due to the attenuation of the electronic buzz; not because of larynx deactivation. At the beginning of the sentence, speech onset is coordinated with activation of the electronic larynx so that the voiced stop /d/ is perceived. This sentence can be heard on the accompanying cassette (Side II, Demonstration D).

Recordings recently were made of two artificial larynx speakers at the University of Florida's Institute for Advanced Study of the Communication Processes. Several clinicians at the Institute and at the Gainesville VA Hospital had classified one speaker as superior and the other as fair to good. Wide-band spectrograms and amplitude displays were made utilizing these recordings, in order to ascertain the aspects of speech signal that provided the basis for the contrasting perceptual judgments of the two speakers. Amplitude measurements of intervocalic stops were made by determining the height of the trace at the end of the preceding vocalic to the peak during the stop-closure. As seen in Figure 9-1, the superior artificial larynx user was able to attenuate the electronic larynx signal by as much as 12 to 18 dB for each of the stop-closures within the sentence. This speaker can be heard on the cassette (Side II, Demonstration D).

An additional difference between the two speakers was that the fair-to-good speaker spoke much more slowly than the superior speaker; primarily because she turned the larynx on and off between words and for stop-closures. These time-consuming actions introduce rhythmic and durational distortions to the speech signal. They also accentuate problems associated with coordinating the electronic larynx buzz for voicing and devoicing. Artificial larynx speakers do not have to produce the completely differentiating characteristics that distinguish voiced and voiceless stop-consonants; rather, these distinctions can be made by varying coupling pressure between the device's vibrating disc and the speaker's neck tissues.

There are many ways of establishing proficiency for turning the device on and off, or attenuating the signal for continuous speech. The method that I least recommend is auditory monitoring with the ear alone, because changes in intensity should and do occur too quickly and subtly to be noticed. Many spectrographs or oscillographs can be used, or if these are not

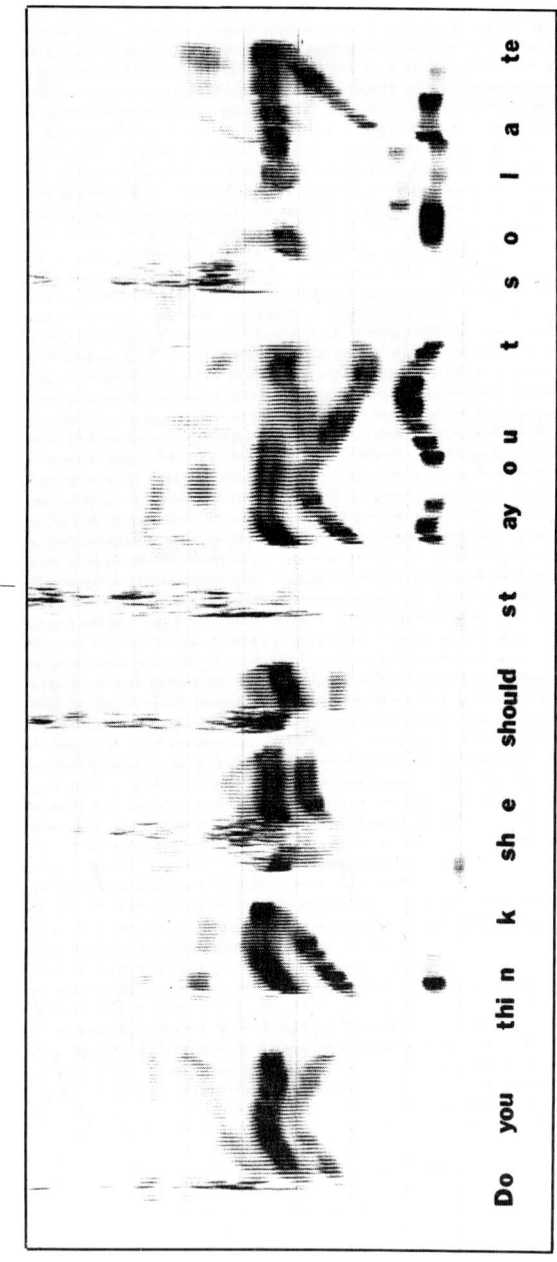

Figure 9-1 (top).

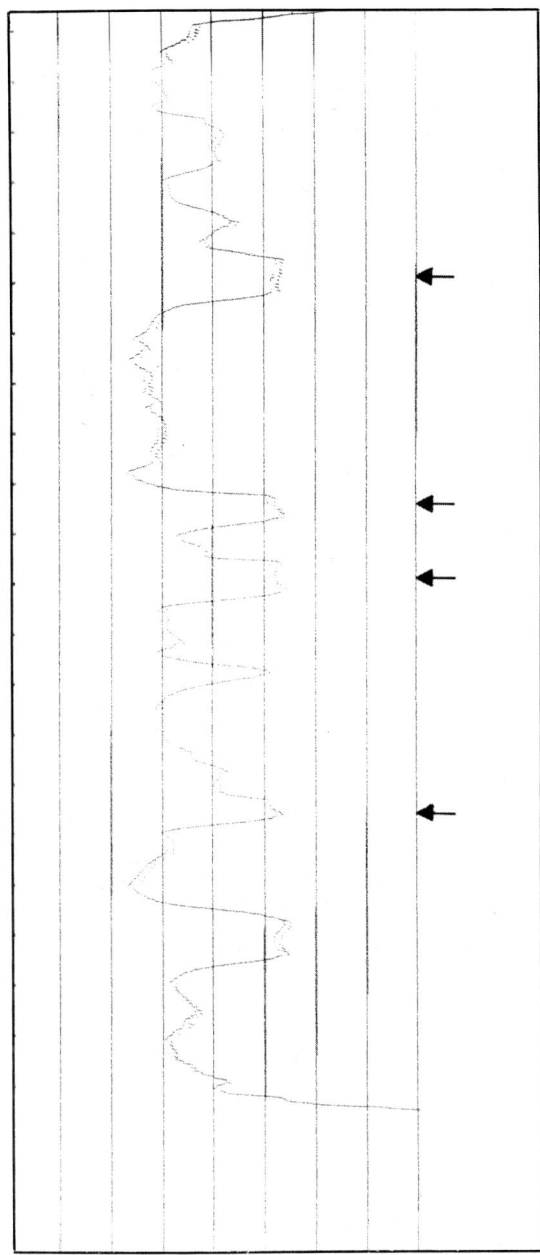

Figure 9-1 (*bottom*). A wideband spectrogram (*top*) and amplitude display (*bottom*) of a superior artificial larynx speaker's production of "Do you think she should stay out so late?" Attenuation of the artificial larynx duty-cycle for the closure of stop consonants is indicated by the arrows at the bottom portion of the figure. The distance between each horizontal line in the amplitude display represents 6 dB.

available, a reel-to-reel tape recorder with edit capabilities or a pause control. Utilizing the edit or pause control leaves the magnetic tape in contact with the play-back head. Slowly moving the tape by hand past the play-back head enables the clinician to hear differences in the intensity of the artificial larynx duty-cycle and time of offset–onset. Through this method, the clinician can also acquire an estimate of the change in intensity by watching the tape recorder VU meter.

As an illustration of this technique, examine Figure 9-1 again. Notice that vertical striations, indicating the electronic larynx duty-cycle, are present throughout the utterance. Attenuation of the duty cycle can be seen by the lightness of the trace during the production of stops and fricatives. These can be measured on the amplitude display. The distance between each horizontal line represents 6 dB. Further, the duration of the attenuation for the stop-closures are appropriate (70 to 90 ms). This example and others can be heard on the cassette (Side II, Demonstration E): measurements of frequency ranges used by the speaker indicate changes up to 80 Hz during the reading of the second sentence from Fairbanks' *Rainbow Passage*,[8] and the eight CID Everyday Sentences utilized by Goldstein and Rothman.[9]

After I met this particular artificial larynx user, I began thinking of her as a virtuoso; she played the electronic larynx with the skill often associated with professional virtuoso musicians. The musical instrument analogy is not far-fetched, as the original artificial larynges used reeds and were based on the same principle as wind instruments. One could observe the quick movements of this speaker's thumb on the pitch control and the subtle hand movements she used at the same time to increase and decrease coupling pressure. All of these movements were rhythmical and coordinated to match the rhythms of her speech.

SUMMARY

I believe that a basic cause of limited speech proficiency with an electronic larynx can be traced to difficulty in appropriate coordination of controls or coupling pressure. Differential manipulations of the electronic larynx in conjunction with the use of buccal air should enable most individuals to attain a high degree of speech intelligibility using most of the artificial larynges currently available.

REFERENCES

1. Stetson RH: Can all laryngectomized patients be taught esophageal speech? Trans Am Laryngol Assoc 59:59–71, 1937
2. Kallen LA: Vicarious vocal mechanisms. AMA Arch Otolaryngol 20:360–503, 1934

3. Morton C: Modern Techniques of Vocal Rehabilitation. Springfield, Charles C Thomas, 1973
4. Isshiki N, Tanabe M: Acoustic and aerodynamic study of a superior electrolarynx speaker. Folia Phoniatr 24:65–76, 1972
5. Lisker L: Closure duration and the intervocalic voiced–voiceless distinction in English. Language 33:42–49, 1957
6. Minifie FD, Hixon TJ, Williams F: Normal Aspects of Speech, Hearing, and Language. Englewood Cliffs, Prentice-Hall, 1973
7. Benguerel AP, Adelman S: Perception of coarticulated lip rounding. Phonetica 33:113–126, 1977
8. Fairbanks G: Voice and Articulation Drillbook (ed 2). New York, Harper & Row, 1960
9. Goldstein LP, Rothman HB: Analysis of speech produced with an artificial larynx. Presented at the American Speech and Hearing Association Convention, Houston, Texas, 1976

Part F

SHIRLEY J. SALMON

Treatment procedures for teaching artificial larynx speech begin the moment that artificial larynges are discussed postoperatively. When speech with an artificial larynx is discussed in a matter-of-fact way, there is no reason to anticipate any attitude other than acceptance by the patient and family members.

Orientation to Artificial Larynges

Most laryngectomized patients feel well enough within five to seven days following surgery to receive a visit from a laryngectomized person who proficiently uses artificial larynx speech. My preference is that the patient receive such a visit prior to a demonstration of all available artificial larynges. Then, when the various types of devices are demonstrated, by me personally or via video-tape, he seems better able to identify with their use.

Prior to a demonstration of the different devices, we adjust the fundamental frequency of each device toward the lower end of the available pitch range. It is necessary to make this adjustment for three reasons. Most artificial larynges are pre-set to produce a fundamental tone higher than the normal male voice. Patients tend to associate their new voices with the first pitch levels used to produce them, and may later resist suggestions to modify the pitch. Finally, we believe that naive users of artificial larynges achieve better resonance, less buzzing, and improved intelligibility with lower pitch levels.

Another suggestion related to pitch adjustment has been made by a patient who interchanges artificial larynx speech and esophageal speech throughout the day. He has adjusted the pitch range on his Western Electric No. 5 so that it approximates the pitch range of his esophageal voice. He reports feeling more comfortable changing from one type of voice to the other when the pitch levels correspond. He also believes that his listeners are more accepting of artificial larynx speech for long periods of time when the fundamental pitch of the device is adjusted toward the lower end of the pitch range.

During the orientation to artificial larynx devices, each instrument is discussed and demonstrated individually. Information is provided about the mechanical parts and how they function, the name and location of the nearest supplier, the purchase price, and finally, the factors related to maintenance and repair. A considerable amount of time is spent in answering questions posed by the patient using a magic slate, and in allowing him both to hold and examine each device.

His curiosity inevitably causes him to want to try producing sound with one or more of the devices. Unless physiological circumstances dictate otherwise, he is encouraged to experiment with the neck-type electronic artificial larynges first; generally, the patient can learn to use them faster than the other types and thus he more rapidly gains the skills necessary for functional communication. Our goal is to help the patient learn to use an artificial larynx well enough to be understood by family members when he is discharged from the hospital. Typically, this must be accomplished within a three-to-four day period.

Placement of the Device

NECK-TYPE DEVICES

The Western Electric No. 5 is recommended initially for trial placement and judgments of resonance potential, because of its lower cost and the convenience of the variable frequency control. Resonance comparable to that achieved with other neck-type electronic larynges usually can be obtained with the Western Electric No. 5 on either side of the neck, under the chin, or on either cheek. Locating the spot for best resonance and determining the most effective coupling are of utmost importance since they are basic to good artificial larynx voice. The clinician should approach these procedures with an experimental attitude and encourage the patient to do likewise. Each time the clinician places the vibrator head on a different location, the on–off tone control must be activated when the patient positions his articulators to produce a vowel, usually *ah*. Judgments of good or poor resonance should then be made by the clinician and patient as varying amounts of coupling pressure are tried. These procedures may be repeated 20 or 30 times before the best resonating spot is determined. (Refer to the accompanying cassette: Side II, Demonstration F.)

Occasionally the Western Electric No. 5 is not a desirable choice. If the patient wears a hearing aid, the vibration from any of the electronic neck-type devices may be amplified and override the patient's speech output, so that self-monitoring is difficult. The Servox seems to cause fewer problems of this type than the Aurex "Neovox" or the Western Electric No. 5, but a mouth-type artificial larynx may prove to be the most satisfactory.

Sometimes acceptable resonance cannot be achieved with the Western Electric No. 5 because:

1. Suture lines are so close together that the vibrating head is too large to couple against the tissue between them.
2. Neck tissue is sensitive to the touch or so firm that only one tiny area is soft enough to permit transmission of sound.
3. The patient has a thin, sometimes short, neck.

When adequate resonance cannot be achieved by neck placement, cheek placement of the Western Electric No. 5 may prove to be adequate. Also, a different electronic neck-type device may provide better resonance.

It is important to note that resonance with an electronic neck-type artificial larynx improves over time even when the most desirable location and effective coupling for acceptable resonance are carefully determined. The location or extent of coupling for best resonance also may change over time. Thus, periodic checks for improved resonance should be made by the clinician and patient as treatment progresses.

MOUTH-TYPE DEVICES

If experimentation with all the electronic neck-type devices fails to yield acceptable resonance, a mouth-type artificial larynx should be considered. We believe that placement of the intra-oral tube is critical for both acceptable resonance and ease of articulation. We instruct the patient to place about $1\frac{1}{2}$ to 2 inches of the intra-oral tube into the side of his mouth and to rest it on the upper lateral surface of his tongue. It is of primary importance that he avoid placing the tube in the mid-line position, which would interfere with production of tongue-tip sounds. Cutting the oral tip of the tube $\frac{1}{4}$-inch in length diagonally and at an approximate 45-degree angle helps to prevent saliva from clogging it. This is especially true when the open side of the slit is placed upward toward the palate.

If the patient is using a mouth-type electronic larynx, we familiarize him with the tone control and then provide instructions about tube placement in the mouth. Similarly, if he is using a pneumatic artificial larynx we instruct him in accurate placement of the stoma cup prior to providing information about tube placement.

Initial Practice in Using the Device

After adequate placement and coupling have been determined, it is necessary to help the patient learn to achieve them accurately and consistently in as short a time as possible. Duguay, Blom, and Goldstein have discussed this topic in their treatment sections of this chapter.

As the patient is learning to achieve adequate resonance, he also can learn to synchronize the tone control with his initiation and termination of vowel productions. Use of a mirror may help him to see that he is activating the tone control prior to assuming the articulatory position appropriate for the vowel he wishes to produce, or vice versa. Similarly, the mirror may show him that he continues to keep the tone control depressed even after he wishes to discontinue phonation; or that he has released the tone control but continues to maintain an articulatory position. It is often more expedient to train the patient to use his auditory feedback system effectively. Generally the patient will learn to control the tone appropriately when:

1. He attempts to synchronize vowel productions with activation and deactivation of the tone control, and carefully attends to visual, auditory, and sensory cues.
2. He makes a judgment of his production.
3. He discusses his judgment with the clinician.
4. He compares his judgment with the clinician's.
5. He accordingly maintains or modifies his behavior during subsequent productions.

We do not believe that the patient must reach 100 percent criterion level with this task prior to beginning more advanced ones. However, because such synchronization is necessary for acceptable artificial larynx speech, he must be made cognizant of the need to perfect this skill.

The patient should be encouraged to maintain a stable frequency level as he learns to produce single vowels intelligibly and to make distinctions between them. Beginning users of artificial larynges often fluctuate from one frequency to another during a single phonation, or from one phonation to the next. This fluctuation should be discouraged since it is distracting to listeners. Later, during the refinement stages, the patient can be taught how to use pitch changes effectively. The patient also should be discouraged from producing stoma noise; it is detrimental both to artificial larynx speech and esophageal speech.

Production of Consonants

When a patient can produce vowels so that listeners can distinguish among them, his practice should take on consonant–vowel combinations with consonants that are not stops or fricatives. The patient subsequently can be instructed to repeat automatic social phrases, to count, to say the days of the week, or to respond to questions for which the answers can be anticipated. These tasks provide the patient practice in applying instructions previously given, and an opportunity to receive reinforcement by the clinician for his efforts to use artificial larynx speech. They also provide the clinician with opportunities to judge overall intelligibility, to listen to the patient's attempts to produce obstruents, and to determine whether any of his behaviors result in involuntary air intake and subsequent esophageal phonation. If the last occurs, the clinician can capitalize on such productions during initial discussions or instructions about air intake for esophageal voice.

We aim for the patient to begin producing meaningful words and phrases prior to his hospital discharge. Although his speech may be grossly intelligible, his difficulty in producing voiced/voiceless distinctions will be noticeably apparent. When he returns as an outpatient to refine his artificial larynx speech and perhaps to begin esophageal speech training, he must learn to compensate for his lack of pulmonary air by modifying his articulation patterns for the production of voiceless stops and fractives. When he can do this, the clinician should begin to listen for voiced/voiceless distinctions. To help the patient acquire these skills, the clinician must provide a simple physiological explanation for why he must do so, some honest feedback, and a few helpful suggestions.

In his treatment section (Chapter 9, p. 129), Goldstein has indicated that direct questions such as "What did you say?" cue the patient that he is not being understood. Specific queries such as "Did you say *pad* or *bad*?" or "Is your wife's name *Sally* or *Ally*?" also emphasize his particular need to utilize oral-pharyngeal pressure for voiceless consonant productions. When the patient is alerted to this need he will typically begin to alter his articulatory patterns. How he achieves such a skill is uncertain. A user of a neck-type device may, as Blom suggests in his treatment section (Chapter 9, p. 121), learn to produce intra-oral-pharyngeal pressure with such intensity that it overrides the voicing inadvertently produced by the artificial larynx. He may, as suggested by Rothman in his treatment section (Chapter 9, p. 133), decrease the coupling pressure of the device, so that the intensity of the tone is decreased and whatever amount of intra-oral-pharyngeal pressure the user creates can be perceived by the listener. Another possibility is that the manipulations described by Rothman result in improved resonance so that the voiceless obstruents can be perceived more readily. A speaker using an intra-oral electronic device may withdraw the mouth tube to a more anterior position to alter resonance, and thus reduce the intensity of the noise source so that intra-oral air pressure is more readily perceived. A speaker using a pneumatic device may utilize oral-pharyngeal air pressure to override the voiced signal. He also might alter the position of his mouth tube to change resonance in a similar way to that described for a user of an intra-oral electronic larynx. Finally, it seems possible that some of these techniques could be combined.

When more explicit instructions are necessary to enable the patient to make distinctions between voice/voiceless consonants, we begin by using an artificial larynx to demonstrate these contrasts in minimal pairs and to help him identify the features that distinguish between "voiced/voiceless obstruents. Sometimes it is necessary to explain that such consonants vary in terms of the turbulence that is associated with voiceless stops and fricatives. To underscore the need for producing turbulence that can be perceived by the listener, practice begins with the patient's production of such consonants without the artificial larynx in position. Then the patient should use his artificial larynx while he practices contrasting voiced/voiceless consonants with a vowel as the clinician provides appropriate feedback. Finally, practice is carried out with minimal paired-word lists that can be conveniently assembled by referring to Fairbanks[1] and Gardner.[2]

The clinician must take a considerable amount of time to encourage the patient to make distinctions between stops and fricatives in the initial position. Patients have to be told and shown how to override a voiced signal or couple the device effectively so that a voiceless consonant can be perceived. Because the /s/ phoneme is especially difficult to produce, patients typically require specific instructions about the articulatory movements they need to perform before it can be perceived accurately. To produce the /s/ phoneme, the patient must use his tongue tip to squeeze intra-oral air against his anterior teeth. He may need considerable practice at producing the /s/ in isolation before he can combine it with other phonemes.

We also encourage our artificial larynx speakers to make voiced/voiceless distinctions of plosives and fricatives in the medial and final position. To do so in the final position, they must terminate their voicing from the device before they release their plosive production, and terminate their voicing from the device before or at the same time they complete their fricative production. For the medial position, we advise them to override their voiced signal or to couple the device effectively so that turbulence can be perceived.

Practice with lists of minimal paired words in which the contrasting consonants occur both in the initial and final positions is also beneficial for the patient's early acquisition of esophageal voice. If the clinician provides esophageal speech training in conjunction with artificial larynx speech training, he or she can often move from teaching voiceless consonants for artificial larynx speech to air injection for esophageal speech.

Refinement Techniques

The overall intelligibility of the patient's speech increases markedly when he has learned to produce obstruents. At that point it will be appropriate to work on phrasing and to encourage a near-normal rate pattern. For more extensive information concerning these topics, refer to the treatment sections by Berry, Blom, Duguay and Goldstein in this chapter.

In the final stages of refinement, instruction should be provided in achieving pitch and loudness changes and when it might be advantageous to utilize them. Loudness of the vibration from neck-type devices can be attenuated by loosening the collar around the vibrating head or by using a thin layer of foam rubber to pad the space around the vibrator. Patients should be encouraged to reduce the loudness of their voices in environments that command an air of quiet reverence, such as in church or at funerals. They should also be made aware of their ability to "whisper" without the aid of a device.

Patients must understand that a decrease in loudness results in the perception of a lowering in pitch and vice versa. Similarly, an increase in loudness results in the perception of a higher pitch, with the reverse phenomenon also true. Thus a patient can communicate increased or decreased loudness and pitch by varying either parameter. All of the ways that he might achieve such modulations are not yet understood but there are several possibilities:

1. He may use the pitch and loudness controls that are available on some of the artificial larynx devices.
2. He may, as Rothman has suggested in his treatment section (Chapter 9, p. 132), vary the extent of coupling pressure.
3. He may alter the resonance cavity by tongue configurations or by tensing his oral-pharyngeal musculature.
4. With a pneumatic device, he may control the amount of pulmonary pressure.

For an example of these techniques, refer to the accompanying cassette (Side II, Demonstration G).

Before a patient can learn to utilize any of these techniques, the clinician must know how the manipulations are performed and be willing to take the time to instruct the patient. However, it is helpful at first to begin working with single vowels or single words. The patient is instructed to produce these utterances at high and low frequency or intensity levels as he experiments with one and later with more of the techniques described previously. When he has begun to feel comfortable with the manipulations, phrases and short sentences can be introduced. Drill on phrases similar to those developed by Fairbanks[1] and Gardner[2] can be utilized to help the patient apply what he has been told or demonstrated.

Some patients will not be able to understand intuitively how to apply these techniques; some will not be able to coordinate the mechanical manipulations; and some will not be motivated to do so. However, other patients will want to learn all they can about artificial larynx devices in order to become proficient speakers with them, and it is these patients for whom refinement techniques should be offered.

I find it useful to provide instruction within a group setting where an exchange of ideas can take place freely and where it is hoped there will be a healthy amount of competition. A group setting also provides an opportunity for reality testing, building of confidence, role playing in short dramatizations, and group singing. It can be a time for fun as well as for learning, and I like to offer it for an hour on a weekly basis. Some of the members of the group have terminated individual treatment but remain active in the group for over a year. Many who are receiving individual therapy for artificial larynx speech and/or esophageal speech elect to attend the group for additional treatment sessions. For whatever needs it fulfills, group therapy is a desirable part of the total treatment program.

ACKNOWLEDGMENT

Throughout this section I have used the term *we* frequently. The choice of the term is deliberate because many people have contributed to the ideas expressed here. Dr. Kay H. Mount, a speech pathologist and speech scientist with whom I have had the pleasure of working, especially deserves credit for her contributions to this section. Without the opportunity to exchange information openly with her and to share experiences that have transpired during treatment sessions, the material presented would be reduced considerably in quantity as well as quality. Her contributions underscore a basic philosophy that inspired the writing of this book. The sharing of ideas advances treatment techniques and, in so doing, improves patient care.

REFERENCES

1. Fairbanks G: Voice and Articulation Drillbook. New York, Harper, 1959
2. Gardner W: Laryngectomee Speech and Rehabilitation. Charles C Thomas, Springfield, 1971

Shirley J. Salmon, Ph.D.

10.
Looking Ahead

The chapters in this book represent opinions from several authors, most of whom have never worked together. The authors are from different geographical areas and their philosophies have evolved from different sets of educational and professional experiences. These experiences have influenced both the type and way that each author has pursued his own clinical and research interests.

Each author for a variety of reasons is interested in the subject of artificial larynx devices, and predictably, each one has investigated the subject in a different way; yet within each chapter are statements similar to those expressed by the other authors here. Superficial consideration of this fact may cause the reader to believe that some of the material is redundant and that the repetitions should have been omitted. With careful reading, however, the reader may conclude, as the editors did, that the repetition reflects a commonality of thought. Such agreement among authors with diverse clinical and research backgrounds is unusual, and we therefore consider it significant enough to emphasize.

All of the contributing authors believe that:

1. Artificial larynx devices should be introduced early in the laryngectomee's speech rehabilitation program.
2. Artificial larynx devices should be selected for individual use based on the patient's needs, skills, preferences, and limitations.
3. Artificial larynx speech should be used first, and later in conjunction with esophageal speech training.
4. Artificial larynx speech is acceptable and the laryngectomee has the right to choose how he will incorporate use of it with his other forms of alaryngeal communication.

None of the authors would deny that there was a time not too long ago when they did not suggest early use of artificial larynges. Nor were they so accepting of patients' decisions to use the devices as a sole means of communication. Even 10 to 15 years ago these ideas were considered ludicrous by most practicing speech–language pathologists. However, ideas accepted on an a priori basis are often altered by a few individualists who speak out against the ideas of the majority.

Professionals such as Heaver,[1] Lueders,[2] Martin,[3] and Miller[4] should be acknowledged for supporting the use of artificial larynges in the early 1950s and late 1960s when it was not popular to do so. But Diedrich and Youngstrom[5] must be given major credit for spear-heading the movement toward more general use and acceptance of artificial larynges. They encouraged use of the devices in the pages of their book, and in the many lectures given by Diedrich throughout the country in the 1960s and early 1970s. Both in the book and in lectures, use of the artificial larynx during the immediate postoperative period was recommended repeatedly. In addition, Diedrich suggested that early use of an artificial larynx would not only satisfy the need for immediate communication, but also would improve the articulatory patterns necessary for the injection method of air intake for esophageal voice. Finally, Diedrich and Youngstrom[5] urged clinicians to recognize the patient's right to choose his own method of alaryngeal communication.

Five years later Gardner[6] reiterated many of the ideas expressed by Diedrich and Youngstrom. He also must be credited with writing the first detailed description of how to conduct speech training with the artificial larynx.

Thus for almost twenty years only a few professionals spoke favorably about use of artificial larynges. More recently, however, increasing numbers of speech-language pathologists have accepted and are encouraging the use of artificial larynges. The effects of their acceptance may be far-reaching and are exciting to think about.

Several modifications of currently available devices have been suggested already. Some of these modifications have been accepted by the manufacturers of artificial larynges and now are incorporated in their newer models. With an increasing number of clinicians and patients using the devices, it seems likely that many more modifications will be suggested in the future. With an increasing demand for devices, it also seems reasonable to expect that current manufacturers will be able to afford to improve their current models and to develop new ones. Further, other people or companies may become involved with designing and distributing new types of alaryngeal devices.

There is little doubt that the increasing interest in artificial larynx speech will initiate more research to explore various facets of it. Such research should provide information that can be utilized to design better devices in terms of speech output, and also in terms of construction, size, ease of operation, and economy. More extensive use of all types of artificial larynges should stimulate interest in determining the acoustic and perceptual characteristics of speech produced with them. It should also result in additional studies being conducted to determine the significant differences between good and poor artificial larynx speech with all types of devices. Selection procedures will become more sophisticated, with recommendations made on the basis of physiological conditions known to affect speech proficiency for each type of device. Treatment procedures should also be researched to delineate those procedures that are unique for each type of artificial larynx.

These are only a few areas to be researched, but the reader can imagine the number of publications that will follow. New information and ideas first will appear in professional journals, and later in publications such as those distributed by the American Cancer Society. The impact of this information on professionals and concerned patients could be most beneficial. It could also be detrimental if we permit our enthusiasm for it to obscure those findings related to all other types of alaryngeal communication. The authors of this book do not wish to encourage such a bias.

We believe that artificial larynx speech should be taught when possible to all laryngectomized individuals who wish to learn it, and that the same should hold true for esophageal speech. We prefer that laryngectomized patients be taught both methods of communication so that they have a choice about when to use one or the other. We hope this handbook contributes much toward the attainment of our goal.

REFERENCES

1. Heaver L, Arnold G: Rehabilitation of alaryngeal aphonia. Post-grad Med 32:11–17, 1962
2. Lueders O: Use of the electrolarynx in speech rehabilitation. AMA Arch Otolaryng 63:133–134, 1956
3. Martin H: Rehabilitation of the laryngectomee. Cancer 16:823–841, 1963
4. Miller M: The responsibility of the speech therapist to the laryngectomized patient. AMA Arch Otolaryng 70:211–216, 1959
5. Diedrich W, Youngstrom K: Alaryngeal Speech. Charles C Thomas, Springfield, 1966
6. Gardner W: Laryngectomee Speech and Rehabilitation. Charles C Thomas, Springfield, 1971

Audio-Cassette Tape Outline

SIDE I

Pneumatic Devices

1. Western Electric 2A
2. Tokyo
3. Osaka
4. Van Human DSP-8
5. Neher 5000

Intra-Oral Electronic Devices

1. Western Electric No. 5, Williams modification
2. Western Electric No. 5, Creech modification
3. Western Electric No. 5, Zwitman modification
4. Cooper-Rand
5. Aurex "Neovox" M-550

Neck-Type Electronic Devices

1. Aurex "Neovox"
2. Barts
3. Servox
4. Western Electric No. 5

Range of Proficiency Demonstrations

A. Speech Projection — M. Duguay

SIDE II

B. On–Off tuning — L. Goldstein
C. Use of Paired Words — L. Goldstein
D. Coordination of Speech and Sound — H. Rothman
E. Attenuation of Sound — H. Rothman
F. Placement — S. Salmon
G. Pitch Changes — S. Salmon

Index

Acoustic cues, 130–131
Acoustic distortions, 131
Acoustic parameters of stop consonant, 131
Acoustic proficiency of artificial larynx speech, 105
Adjusting pitch of artificial larynx, 137–138
Aerodynamic proficiency of artificial larynx speech, 105
Air bypass speech and esophageal speech
 acceptability, 80–81
 acoustic features, 80–81
 comparison of, 79–81
 duration, 80–81
 intelligibility, 80–81
 rate, 80–81
American Cancer Society, 45
Arnold GE, 57
Arslan M, 79
Arthritis, see Dexterity
Articulation
 analysis of, 94–110
 in artificial larynx speech, 121
 poor habits, 24
Artificial larynx
 adjusting pitch of, 137–138
 advantages of, 13
 age as a factor, 14
 bias against, 17, 40, 116
 calling attention to, 12
 clinicians' lack of experience with, 40
 clinicians' lack of training with, 44
 decisions for issuing, 14
 demonstration of, 137
 disadvantages of, 11–12
 growing acceptance of, 146
 handling of, 13
 importance of proper instruction, 14
 improving articulation and intelligibility, 8
 mechanical adjustments, 119–200
 mechanical quality, 117

151

Artificial larynx (*continued*)
  modifications of, 146–147
  monotonous sound of, 122
  orientation to, 138
  placement of, 120, 125, 138–139
  presentation of, 127–128
  proficiency of communication, 29
  reasons for making available, 15
  reducing tension and anxiety, 8
  selection of, 123, 132
  sign of defeat, 12
  speech, 89
  teaching advantages to laryngectomee, 14–15
  to facilitate development of esophageal speech, 7–8
  used by esophageal speakers, 117
  used to break faulty habits, 8
Artificial larynx speakers
  emotional reactions, 46
  instruction for use of device, 47
  introduction to device, 45
  introduction to esophageal speech, 45
  respondent, 44
  survey of, 44–45
  types of devices, 46
  visitations, 45
Artificial larynx speech
  accurate onset of voicing, 120
  articulation, 121
  attenuation, 133–136
  evaluation of, 87–110
  extraneous noise, 94
  frequency of, 91–94
  varying pitch and intensity, 122, 132, 143–144
Artificial larynx speech and esophageal speech
  advantages of using both, 9
  choosing one, 8–9, 18
  comparison of, 27–28
  taught simultaneously, 6
Asai R, 79
Attitudes
  how it will influence choice, 22
  how they are transmitted, 5
  of otolaryngologists, 35–39, 40
  of speech pathologists, 40
  ways to improve, 48
Audio-visual, 28
Auditory monitoring, 21
Aurex "Neovox," 46, 62, 77–78, 91, 94, 105, 123, 139
Aurex "Neovox" M-550, 71–72

Bailey B J, 89
Bardner, 142
Barts Vibrator Electronic Larynx, 75–77
Behavior modification in rehabilitation, 116–117
Bennett S, 28, 29, 92
Bias
  against artificial larynx, 17, 116
  against quality of artificial larynx speech, 40
  prevention of, 18–19
  toward esophageal speech, 43–44
Billroth, 57, 58, 89
Blom ED, 80
Brucke, 58
Bruns P, 59
Buccal air
  and voiceless stop, 132–133
  in articulation, 98
  in treatment, 132–133
  need for, 132–133

Cannula
  flexible, 59
  laryngeal, 58, 59
  phonatory, 58

INDEX 153

tracheal, 58, 60
Clinicians
  lack of experience with artificial larynx, 40
  lack of training with artificial larynx, 44
Closure duration in artificial larynx speech, 104
Coarticulation, 131
Cognates, 129, 130, 138, 142
  producing contrast of, 105, 121
Communication
  defined, 4, 5
  expanded with artificial larynx, 8
  need for, 4
  perception of, 130–131
  proficiency, 29
Cooper HK, 61, 62
Cooper-Rand Electronic Speech Aid, 46, 66–68, 72, 123
Cost (influencing choice of device), 23
Counseling
  factors to be covered, 19–20
  importance of, 18
  presentation of information, 20
  prevention of bias, 18–19
Conley JJ, 79
Consistency of placement
  making of area for placement, 125, 128
  use of mirror, 128
Creech modification, 68
Crouse GP, 28, 32
Curry ET, 92
Czermak JN, 53, 54, 55

Danapipe, 62
Danavox International, 62
Demonstrations of artificial larynx, 137
Dentures, 21

Dexterity (influencing choice of device), 22
Diedrich WM, 12, 146
Disadvantages of artificial larynx, 11–12
Dutch DSP8, 123
Dysarthria, 21

Early treatment and selection of device, 117
Edwards N, 79
Electronic artificial larynx, 28, 32, 57, 60, 62, 66–79
  mouth-type devices, 66–72
    Aurex Neovox M-550, 71–72
    Cooper-Rand Electronic Speech Aid, 66–68
    Modified Western Electric No. 5, 68–71
    Ticchioni Pipe, 72
    Verbalizer Voice Synthesizer, 72
  neck-type devices, 72–79
    Aurex "Neovox," 77–78
    Barts Vibrator Electronic Larynx, 75–77
    Servox, 78–79
    Western Electric 5A and 5B, 72–75
Environment (influencing choice of device), 22
Electromagnetically activated artificial larynx, 61
Esophageal speech
  acceptability, 4
  artificial larynx as an aid to, 143
  bias for, 39, 43–44
  developing a higher level of proficiency, 7
  percent of failure, 5
  quality of, 6
  selection of, 4

Esophageal speech and air bypass speech, *see* Air bypass speech and esophageal speech
Esophageal speech and artificial larynx speech, *see* Artificial larynx speech and esophageal speech
Evaluating artificial larynx speech, 87–110
Extraneous noise in artificial larynx speech, 94

Fairbanks G, 121, 122, 142, 144
Feedback, 129
Fisher HB, 4
Flexible cannula, 59
Fould, 59
Frequency analysis of artificial larynx speech, 91–94
Fricatives
  duration of, 97
  in analysis of artificial larynx speech, 104
  in articulation of artificial larynx speech, 97, 121, 142
  in artificial larynx speech, 110
  in characteristics of artificial larynx speech, 105
  voiceless, 95
Fundamental skills of artificial larynx user, 118–119

Gardner WN, 5, 144, 146
Goldstein LP, 29, 32, 45, 90, 136
Goode RL, 119
Gottstein G, 60
Gluck T, 59, 60, 61
Group setting advantages, 144
Gussenbauer C, 58

Hanson WL, 57
Hearing (influencing choice of device), 21

Heaver L, 146
Hochenegg J, 59
Horn D, 5
Hyman M, 27

Inflection, 121, 122
Intelligibility, 12, 28, 32, 80–81, 123, 130–131
  achieving normal rate of speech with artificial larynx, 129
  comparison of artificial larynx speech and esophageal speech, 27–40
Intensity analysis of artificial larynx speech, 84, 91
Intervocalic plosive, 133
Intra-oral electronic larynx indications, 21
Irvine, 59
Isshiki N, 94, 105, 110, 121, 130

Kalb MB, 29, 32
Kallen LA, 57, 58, 130
Kett Mark III, 46, 62
King PS, 5
Knepflar K, 48
Knox A, 48
Knox modification, 70
Komorn RM, 79

La Barge Voice Bak, 80
Laryngectomee
  dissatisfaction with artificial larynx, 13
  needs of, 4
  return to employment, 14
  use of artificial larynx, 7
Laryngectomee Club, 9
  Lost Voice Club of Cleveland, 9
  New Voice Club, 43
Laryngeal cannula, 58, 59
Laryngeal stenosis, 58
Laryngo-pharyngectomy, 81
Lauder E, 15

INDEX

Lebrun Y, 57, 62
Leiter J, 58, 59
"Lending Bank," 123
Lions Club, 123
Listener judgment, 32
Listener preference of alaryngeal
 speech, 28
Logemann J, 83
Loudness, 27
Lueders O, 146

McCroskey R, 28, 32
MacKenty, 60
McKesson E, 60
Martin H, 5, 60, 146
Mechanical adjustments of arti-
 ficial larynx, 119–120
Mechanical quality of artificial
 larynx, 117
Miller M, 146
Modifications of alaryngeal
 devices, 146–147
Modified surgical esophagostomy,
 79
Modified Western Electric No. 5,
 68–71
 Creech Modification, 68
 Knox Modification, 70–71
 Williams and Ostroy Modifica-
  tion, 69–70
 Zwitman and Disinger Mod-
  ification, 70
Monotonous sound of artificial
 larynx, 122
Montgomery WW, 79
Morton C, 130
Mouth-type devices, 58–73,
 139–140

Neck tissue, 17–22
Neck-type artificial larynx, 73–79,
 89, 141, 138–139, 143
 hand preference, 124
 placement, 124

 transcervical and throat type,
  58
Neher 5000 Artificial Larynx, 66
Normal speech production, 87–89
Northwestern Voice Prosthesis,
 82–84

Onodi, 60
Oral habits (influencing choice of
 device), 21
Oral hygiene, 21
"Oral Vibrator," 62
Orientation to artificial larynx,
 138
Osaka (Yamamura), 46, 65
Otolaryngologists
 attitudes of, 35–39
 cooperation with speech
  pathologists, 41

Patient's right to choose, 146
Perception of communication,
 130–131
Phonemes, 105, 131, 142
Phrasing in artificial larynx
 speech, 121, 126
Phonatory cannula, 58
Pilcher H, 61
Pitch and loudness
 varying in artificial larynx,
  143–144
 with pneumatic artificial larynx,
  120, 122
Pitch variation in Western Electric No. 5, 122
Placement of artificial larynx
 drills, 120, 128
 for best resonance, 138–139
 on an individual with a hearing
  aid, 125
 use of mirror in, 125
Plosives, 95, 142
Plosive energy in artificial larynx
 speech, 105

Plosive noises in artificial larynx speech, 121
Pneumatic artificial larynx, 27, 32, 57–60, 63–66, 119, 120, 122, 123, 140, 142
  description of, 63–66
  development of, 58
  Neher 5000, 66
  Osaka, 65
  pitch and loudness variability, 120, 122
  placement of, 120
  Tokyo, 63–65
  Van Humen, 66
Postoperative
  fistula, 21
  how artificial larynx helps, 6
  visit by laryngectomee, 137
Presentation of artificial larynx to laryngectomee, 127–128
Putney EJ, 5

Quality of artificial larynx, 123

Rate, 27, 28, 91–93, 121, 129
Rating attitudes, 37
Reed–fistula method
  intelligibility, 81–82
  frequency, 82
  phonation time, 82
Reed material (metal and rubber), 59
Rehabilitation team, 18
Reisz RR, 60
Resonance, 142
Refinement techniques
  pitch, 143–144
  loudness changes, 143–144
Reynaud, 57
Role of therapist for decision making, 5
Rotary Club, 123
Rothman HB, 94

Selection
  of artificial larynx devices, 21–23, 123, 132
  of artificial larynx versus esophageal speech, 4, 8–9, 18
  patient's right to choose, 146
  of listeners, 32
Sentence intelligibility, 28
Serafini I, 79
Sertoma Club, 123
Servox Electronic Larynx, 46, 78–79, 139
Shames GH, 28
Shedd D, 79, 81
Shipp T, 92
Sisson GA, 79, 82–84
Sonovox, 62
Speech communication (determining proficiency)
  articulation, 94–110
  frequency, 91, 92
  intensity, 93–94
  rate, 92–93
Speech pathologists
  and otolaryngologists cooperation, 41
  attitudes of, 35, 39–40
  judgments to be avoided by, 124
Speech production, 88
  alternate modes of, 87
Speech proficiency parameters, 110
Stetson RH, 130
Stoma cup placement, 140
Stoma phobia influencing choice of device, 22
Stop-closure duration, 95
Stop release in artificial larynx articulation, 105
Stork, 59
Stress, 121–122

Surgery influencing choice of device, 21
Surgical prosthetics, 79–84

Tait V, 61–62
Tait Oral Vibrator, 121
Tape recorder for timing artificial larynx speech, 121
Tapia A, 60
Taub S, 79
Tel-Communication, 117
Temporal distortions, 131
Ticchioni Pipe, 72
Timing, 120–121
Tokyo artificial larynx, 29, 46, 63–65, 81
Tracheal cannula, 58, 60
Treatment
  acceptance of laryngectomee, 127–128
  altering articulatory patterns, 141
  approaches, 115–147
  avoiding artificiality, 132
  behavioral modification, 116–117
  compensation for pulmonary air, 141
  consistency of placement, 128, 129
  controlling voicing mechanism, 132
  developing adequate buccal pressure, 132
  for maximum listener ability, 131–132
  group setting, 144
  maintaining stable frequency level, 140
  need for further research, 147
  production of consonants, 141

refinement techniques, 143
selection of proper device, 117
summary of authors' views, 145–146
synchronizing tone control, 140
use of non-dominant hand, 124, 128
Trial aids influencing choice of device, 23
Turbulence, 142

Van Humen artificial larynx, 66
Vega MF, 79
Verbalizer Voice Synthesizer, 72, 73
Vocalics, 95
Voice-voiceless, see Cognates
Vocophone, 60

Weinberg B, 81
Western Electric No. 1, 60
Western Electric No. 2, 29, 60, 61
Western Electric No. 5, 29, 46, 72–75, 91, 92, 119, 122, 123, 138
  modification to battery compartment, 75–76
  pitch adjustment, 74
  problems with resonance, 139
  training how to vary pitch, 126
Williams and Ostroy modification, 69
Wireless induction system, 61
Wolff J, 59
Word intelligibility, 28
Wright, 62

Yamamura, see Osaka

Zwitman and Disinger modification, 70